Using CBT and Mindfulness to Manage Student Anxiety

Using CBT and Mindfulness to Manage Student Anxiety provides a weekly framework utilizing cognitive behavioral therapy and mindfulness to support children who are struggling with anxiety.

This book begins with an overview of cognitive-behavioral therapy (CBT) and mindfulness practices and their use in supporting worry. The 9 weekly sessions are broken down into a ready-to-use lesson complete with an assessment tool, clinician notes for added depth, and a template to support generalization of learning with teachers and guardians. Lessons are focused on connection, building an awareness of emotions, and increasing the student's capacity to regulate their emotions in a variety of ways. The last portion of this book offers opportunities to continue generalization of emotion regulation skills in the classroom and at home.

Providing practitioners with a ready-to-go structured lesson plan that builds with each session, and tools to assess progress and growth, this book will be a welcome addition to any school-based mental health professional's library.

Katelyn Oellerich, EdS, is a nationally certified school psychologist practicing in Wisconsin. In 2022, Katelyn was recognized as the Wisconsin School Psychologist of the Year.

"Anxiety can be so tricky, yet Katelyn puts together a practical and well laid out guide (or curriculum) to support tweens and teens to address it head on. Weaving together mindfulness and CBT into 9 lessons, teachers and clinicians will be well equipped to teach adolescents multiple strategies to manage their anxiety with ease."

Leah Kuypers, MA Ed., OTR/L, *creator and author of* The Zones of Regulation

"Katelyn Oellerich's book, *Using CBT and Mindfulness to Manage Student Anxiety,* will be an enormous help to school psychologists and school counselors who are looking to use a manual for a group or individual intervention for students struggling with anxiety related difficulties. From scripted openings to sessions and discussion prompts, to great handouts, figures and 'how to' directions, this book will answer the question, 'where can I begin and what should I include' in a helpful anxiety & coping skill intervention for students. Keep this book in your school mental health library for practitioners."

Rebecca Comizio, *co-author of the* Resilience Workbook for Kids, *nationally certified school psychologist & licensed professional counselor*

"In this valuable book, Katelyn offers not only a warning but research-based advice about practices that she has seen make a difference with young people experiencing worry, anxiety and trauma. It's an excellent resource for counselors, advisory leaders, and school administrators who want to understand more about the best ways to help students survive and thrive in increasingly difficult times."

John Norton, *founder & co-editor, MiddleWeb.com*

"Over the past few years, schools have become the primary source of support for students in a time of significant social and societal disruption and change. This curriculum offers a well-researched formula for supporting students who experience symptoms and feelings of anxiety as a result. Most importantly, it provides clear and easy-to-use lesson plans and scripts for clinicians who are most often on the frontlines of supporting students through emotions that can disrupt or impede their ability to fully exist in the world."

Abby Morrison, *school social worker*

Using CBT and Mindfulness to Manage Student Anxiety

A 9-Week Program for Children and Adolescents

Katelyn Oellerich, EdS

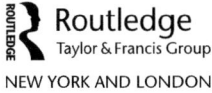
Routledge
Taylor & Francis Group

NEW YORK AND LONDON

Cover image: © Getty Images

First published 2023
by Routledge
605 Third Avenue, New York, NY 10158

and by Routledge
4 Park Square, Milton Park, Abingdon, Oxon, OX14 4RN

Routledge is an imprint of the Taylor & Francis Group, an informa business

ISBN: 978-1-032-34991-6 (hbk)
ISBN: 978-1-032-34990-9 (pbk)
ISBN: 978-1-003-32478-2 (ebk)

DOI: 10.4324/9781003324782

Typeset in ITC New Baskerville Std
by KnowledgeWorks Global Ltd.

I would like to dedicate this book to a number of special people that have inspired and supported me along the way.

- My students, past and present that continue to show up even when life feels tough.
- The amazing co-workers, families, and community members I've had the privilege of learning from.
- My parents, who taught me how to believe in change and in myself.
- My husband, who has helped me in every idea and project I've dreamt up.

And mostly, this book is dedicated to my children, who inspire my work to support mental health daily.

Contents

Foreword   ix

Acknowledgments   x

About the Author   xi

1 The Presentation of Worry and Anxiety in Children and Adolescents   1

What Is Worry? 2
How Is Worry Different from Anxiety? 2

2 What Is Cognitive Behavioral Therapy?   7

Emotions, Thoughts, and Behaviors 8
Reframing Thoughts 10
What Is Within Our Control and What Is Out of Our Control? 15
Coping Strategies 17
CBT Conclusion 19

3 How Can Mindfulness Support CBT?   21

What Is Mindfulness? 21
How to Cultivate Mindfulness 22
Emotion Awareness 23
Mindfulness and CBT 23

4 How to Use this Book   29

Student Selection 29
Strategies Utilized in Chapters 5–15 29
Chapters 5–13 Explained 30
Chapter 14 Explained 31
Chapter 15 Explained 31

5 Week 1: Introduction/Get to Know Each Other   33

Week 1 Outline 33
Week 1 Clinician Notes 35
Teacher and Guardian Summary 39

6 Emotions   41

Week 2 Outline 41
Week 2 Clinician Notes 43
Teacher and Guardian Summary 45

7 Our Body and Our Thoughts   47

Week 3 Outline 47
Week 3 Clinician Notes 50
Teacher and Guardian Summary 53

8 Changing Thoughts and Working through Problems   55

Week 4 Outline 55
Week 4 Clinician Notes 60
Teacher and Guardian Summary 63

9 In and Out of Control/Coping Strategies   65

Week 5 Outline 65
Week 5 Clinician Notes 67
Teacher and Guardian Summary 69

10 People That Help Our Thoughts   71

Week 6 Outline 71
Reference to Appendix K 72
Session 10 Clinician Notes 74
Teacher and Guardian Summary 76

11 Coping Strategies   79

Session 11 Outline 79
Session 11 Clinician Notes 82
Teacher and Guardian Summary 84

12 Student Plan   85

Session 8 Outline 85
Week 8 Clinician Notes 88
Teacher and Guardian Summary 90

13 Completion/Next Steps   91

Session 9 Outline 91
Session 9 Clinician Notes 93
Teacher and Guardian Summary 94

14 Continued Support for the Classroom   97

Emotions Check-in 98
Calm Space 101
Daily Mindfulness 104
Short Mindful Moments 109
Deep Breathing Graphics 110
Accommodations 113
Individualized Education Plan (IEP) Goals 115

15 Continued Support for Home   117

Gratitude Reflection 118
Calm Space 121
Family Mindfulness 123
A Worry Box 125
What Went Well Today 126
Specific Praise Each Night 127
What Is Something You're Looking Forward to Today? 128

Appendices   131
Index   150

Foreword

If you're looking at this book, you're probably concerned about how to help your students cope with anxiety and stress. You may already know something about CBT and may even use CBT-based approaches in your work with students. You may be familiar with mindfulness or even practice mindfulness in your own life. But, you may also be struggling with how to best put research and theory into practice with your students. This book could be a valuable resource for you. It is a "how to" guide for the busy school-based professional looking for a plan that integrates varied methods from existing CBT and mindfulness approaches. You'll likely see some methods that you already know and use. And, you're also likely to find some strategies that are new to you. However, I think the thing you'll like best is having multiple resources and strategies organized for you in one volume. You'll find screening and assessment measures, worksheets for students, information for the adults in their lives, and a weekly session plan that links all of this information together in one place.

As a professor it's always a joy to see students excelling as professionals. When I knew Katelyn many years ago in our School Psychology program, I valued her thoughtful and organized approach to school psychology. That organizational clarity and thoughtfulness is one of the greatest strengths of this book. For those who need a refresher on theory and research, the early chapters give you an overview of theory and research on anxiety and worry, the cognitive-behavioral model, and mindfulness approaches. This review information is made more accessible through the use of case examples. I appreciated the clarification of her case conceptualization examples and can see myself sharing that with graduate students.

If your focus is more on "how do I do this," you'll head right to Chapters 5 through 13 where she takes you through the nine sessions of her intervention plan. In each chapter, you'll find an outline stating session goals and needed materials, followed by specific activities, suggested wording, and "clinician notes" to facilitate your work. As with most CBT approaches, you'll find sessions focused on emotions, thinking, and problem-solving. In this book, you'll also find a session focused on relationships (e.g., people who help), which is less commonly seen in discussions of CBT with youth. And, to help you pull it all together, in Chapter 12, you'll find clear guidance on helping your student create an individual "worry plan."

As school professionals, one of your concerns is helping students to use skills and cope effectively in a range of settings, not just the therapy office. In Chapters 13 and 14, you'll find information and strategies to share with the adults in your students' lives – their teachers and guardians. There are specific explanations of strategies for adults to provide additional supports at home and in the classroom. As with all of the chapters, the focus is on practical implementation, with specific instructions and materials that you can make your own, for your students.

I look forward to turning to this book as I teach graduate students to practice CBT. I anticipate recommending it as a resource for many!

Barbara R. Beaver, Ph.D.
Professor, Department of Psychology
University of Wisconsin-Whitewater

Acknowledgments

The process of writing this book involved support from many people. I would like to thank my friends and colleagues, Jenny Singer and Danielle Swenson, and school psychologist and cohort friend, Amanda Palmer, for providing helpful feedback on my book outline and planning of this book. My principal and fellow author, Matt Renwick, for supporting me in the process of writing my first book. He helped to guide and mentor me through the navigation of publication. I would also like to thank John Norton, creator of Middle Web, for allowing me the chance to try my hand at writing for a large audience and connecting me with this opportunity.

I next want to thank my friend, Christy Hamilton Cole, for her support in reading over this book and providing feedback to clarify the text and make it not only clinician friendly but also child friendly. Her willingness to support this endeavor is incredibly appreciated. Also, to the group that introduced me to Christy and gave me the courage to believe in my dreams, Compounding Courage. To all of you strong humans, thank you for showing up on Saturday mornings to support courageous thinking. Your support and compassion could truly move mountains.

Finally, I'd like to acknowledge the support of my professors at the University of Wisconsin-Whitewater, especially Dr. Barbara Rybski Beaver, for guiding and propelling me forward through many varying life stages and pushing me constantly to be a better writer and psychologist.

About the Author

Katelyn Oellerich, EdS, is in her 9th year as a practicing school psychologist. She was recognized as the Wisconsin School Psychologist of the Year in 2022. Katelyn has a passion for supporting student needs and helping to generalize that learning with families and in the classroom. Katelyn lives in the country with her husband and two kids.

1 The Presentation of Worry and Anxiety in Children and Adolescents

Worry … it's something we all experience from time to time. It can be described as that feeling you get when you can't remember if you turned off the stove before you left and you are an hour from home. Or the experience of arriving at the airport late and realizing you have five minutes to make it to your gate. Worry is felt when your loved one is late getting home and isn't answering their phone.

Worry is a common concern that arises in all of us and can especially be obvious in students who are school aged. It seems that as kids begin to grow and become adolescents, there is an additional pressure put on them for meeting social norms, being involved in a multitude of activities, excelling in school, and meeting parent expectations. In addition to these worries that can come up for all children, some kids may also worry about how their family will pay for certain necessities, where they will be sleeping for that night, what they will eat, who will be taking care of them, or how safe their home is feeling.

The feeling of worry is relative to the individual person. Each of us has influences that may increase worry in our lives as well as resiliency factors. Resiliency involves the skills to adapt to tough life experiences through mental, emotional, and behavioral flexibility as well as the capacity to be flexible and adjust to internal and external demands (American Psychological Association, 2012). Factors that contribute to resiliency include a person's view of and interaction with the world, resources including access to basic needs, and coping mechanisms (American Psychological Association, 2012). A person's access to resiliency factors may impact how they respond to stress and, in turn, how they experience worry. Take for instance the example of someone whose car just broke down on the side of the road. This can be a stressful situation for anyone. A person who broke down in an area in which they feel safe, has access to resources such as family or friends who can come to help, and has money set aside to support them in emergencies is going to feel less long-lasting stress and worry from this event. However, a person who breaks down in an area where they do not feel safe, has limited access to resources including a lack of family and friends willing to support, and is lacking financial resources to help in an emergency is going to feel more long-lasting stress and worry from this event.

Another way in which resiliency factors can be broken down is by considering a person's temperament. Attitude and openness to express emotions can impact overall resiliency (Smith Harvey, 2007). A child with a more positive outlook and openness to experiences may recognize that it's raining outside and express disappointment over not being able to play basketball like they planned during recess but also look forward to a different activity inside with friends, whereas a child with less resiliency and openness to change may view rain negatively and become very upset and struggle to see the positive in an alternative option, missing most of their recess time due to difficulty in regulating their feelings.

With children and adolescents spending a lot of their time in the school setting, school staff are given a unique opportunity to support building resiliency within students. Research has shown that

DOI: 10.4324/9781003324782-1

schools can promote resiliency by building relationships with students, empowering students, and supporting students (Rose & Steen, 2014). Staff can support building relationships through regular emotion check-ins each day, mentoring relationships, and peer support groups. Empowerment can be encouraged by reinforcing behavior, "You are working so hard on that worksheet, way to persevere!" rather than praising the student themselves, "You are so smart!" Support of coping strategies can also be taught and normalized across the school system.

What Is Worry?

For this book, worry is defined as when the mind is focused on something and continues to perseverate on that thought and get caught in the negative. People worry about many different things including something that could happen like failing a test or something that has already happened like tripping in front of friends. Worry often involves the mind getting stuck on an idea and can negatively impact thoughts and behavior. However, worry can also be helpful at times because it can support preparation for future danger (Mathews, 1990). Worry becomes a problem when it occurs frequently and impacts the ability to follow through with actions (Mathews, 1990). Worry can influence the mind's capacity to think about anything outside of what is causing the feeling of worry. When this happens, thoughts can become stuck, and it can be challenging to work through certain activities.

Research has shown that the less control we have in a situation, the more worry we tend to feel (Sacco & Glackman, 1987). In general, for kids, there are certain things they know they need to do whether they want to or not: go to school, share a home with their family, complete homework, and follow their parent's rules. When these tasks are not done, there is usually a consequence. Therefore, it is not surprising that when situations arise that feel out of control, our children and adolescents may especially struggle because they have so few choices already.

How Is Worry Different from Anxiety?

Anxiety differs from worry in that people with anxiety tend to avoid situations where they may feel anxious, they experience intense fear, and they worry much more than is expected about typical stressors (Cleveland Clinic, 2017). Some worry can be expected from all people at some points in time; however, it becomes problematic when it begins to impact daily living. A child who experiences worry during storms may have some of their thoughts consumed when it is thundering outside. Whereas a child with anxiety about storms will be unable to focus whenever the clouds begin to darken, struggles to sleep when it is raining, and constantly finds themselves thinking about what may happen when it storms.

Some children and adolescents may be able to name their feelings and recognize maladaptive thoughts as problematic. However, many children and adolescents need further support in identifying how they are holding onto their anxiety. Symptoms of anxiety can present in three different ways: physically (e.g., headaches, stomachaches, racing heart), behaviorally (e.g., avoidance of certain activities), and cognitively (e.g., negative thinking patterns, difficulty focusing) (Cleveland Clinic, 2017).

Physical Symptoms

Physical Symptoms have been found to be highly related to overall well being and self-perception (Lieutaud, Grenier, & Bois, 2021). Some physical symptoms can help in preparation for a tough situation. For instance, an increased heart rate can ready the body for the need to run away. Body signals can also serve as a reminder to check in with our thoughts and feelings. For example, my stomach doesn't feel well, why might that be? Oh yes, I just was reminded about the test we have tomorrow that I don't feel prepared to take.

Although physical symptoms can serve a useful purpose, research indicates that holding onto body sensations related to anxiety can actually lead to more anxiety in the future (Dijkstra-Kersten et al., 2015) Therefore, awareness of physical symptoms is crucial in supporting next steps toward recognizing and accepting emotions that arise and change. Recognizing the clues from the body involves observing the state of the body when feeling calm and then noticing what occurs differently within the body once that feeling is shifted. The following are examples of some physical symptoms that may accompany somatic complaints:

- Rapid heart rate.
- Stomachache.
- Headache.
- Sweaty hands.
- Flushed cheeks.

Some people who experience physical symptoms related to anxiety struggle to make the connection between their physical pain, thoughts, and emotions. In these cases, it is especially important to take the time to talk through how anxiety feels for them. This can be done by breaking down what happened prior to the symptom, what thoughts arose, and what feelings were noticed.

Cognitive Symptoms

Minahan and Rappaport (2012) propose that students with anxiety may have underdeveloped skills in the following areas:

- Self-regulation: being able to manage intense emotions.
- Thought stopping: worry tends to lead to concerns for the worst-case scenario and thinking more negatively.
- Thinking traps: an ability to recognize and manage common patterns in thinking that can lead to increased anxiety.
- Social skills: being able to recognize another's perspective and respond accordingly.
- Executive functioning: thinking about the consequences of actions and being able to follow the steps necessary to complete a task.
- Flexible thinking: the ability to be able to shift thinking and consider alternative options and viewpoints to problems.

These lagging skills can impact overall thought processes. Knowing that students with anxiety are lacking in some or all of these skills provides a framework of how to support thought development and reduce anxiety.

Behavioral Symptoms

Anxiety also can impact behaviors. Anxiety is often related to behaviors of avoidance. People with anxiety tend to be more likely to be concerned with the risk of something negative happening in a situation and therefore are less likely to take a risk (Maner & Schmidt, 2006). Pittig et al. (2021) further explained that even when something pleasurable is offered, if a threat of risk is indicated, those individuals struggle to inhibit their avoidance response and tend to continue to avoid the situation. Avoided experiences are unique to each individual but could include avoiding going to a party, going on a trip, or trying something new.

Case Studies

The feeling of anxiety is uncomfortable and can influence how a person acts with an intent to reduce or rid themselves of that feeling of worry. As a way to better understand and consider anxiety, four students with different types of anxiety will be discussed. The following case studies will begin by describing the students.

Braden – Phobia of Germs

Braden is a student who is in fifth grade. Braden is wonderful at math, enjoys playing basketball and baseball, and is part of the choir. This year lots of people have been getting sick, and Braden is finding it harder and harder to focus on his schoolwork. If Braden hears another person cough or blow their nose, he becomes worried that he is going to get their sickness. Braden's teachers have noted the change in his behavior, explaining he can be easily distracted and often seems on edge. Braden enjoys being creative, especially when he has the chance to write or draw about superheroes.

Mari – Separation Anxiety

Mari is a fourth-grade student who recently lost her dad. Mari just moved to a new town with her mom and two sisters. Mari is well-liked by the other students and received lots of compliments for her performance at the talent show. Mari also has solid academic skills across all areas and sometimes serves as a tutor for other kids in the class who need more help. However, Mari often expresses worrying about her mom when she is not with her. Mari sometimes cries during class and has a hard time focusing on her work during any independent time because she wants to make sure that her mom is ok. She shares feelings of concern for something happening to her mom when she is not with her, especially when she is expected to work on her own or quietly. Mari is able to feel most calm after talking to someone who can support her in bringing her thoughts back to more likely scenarios (e.g., mom is most likely safe and ok right now) as well as having that person to support her in calming herself with relaxation strategies. Mari has also reported feeling some relief in worries when she is able to do something that involves physical activity.

Juliana – Generalized Anxiety

Juliana is a straight A student in sixth grade. She is involved in sports, clubs, and works a part-time job babysitting after school. Juliana has high expectations for herself and has been described as becoming very upset if things are not in perfect order. Juliana's dad has shared that one time her family helped to put away one of her blankets and they didn't fold it correctly, so she began to get very upset. Juliana yelled, paced, and sat in the corner of her room and picked at the carpet. The only way that Juliana could feel better is to fix the blanket. Juliana's father also explained that she is often up late at night doing laundry. Juliana shared that her mind feels most calm when she's listening to meditative practices that guide her thoughts to focus on her breath and being in the moment.

Janarion – Significant Somatic Symptoms and Social Anxiety

Janarion is an eighth-grade student. Janarion often has stomachaches and misses a lot of school. He rarely talks at school, but at home his parents describe him as being very talkative. Janarion often goes to see the nurse for stomachaches. In the classroom, it is hard for Janarion to focus on the lesson and his parents have explained that he feels the room is too noisy and he doesn't want the teacher to call on him. Janarion's parents have also expressed that at home they don't talk much about emotions, and teach their children the importance of "sucking it up." Janarion spends most of his days attempting to avoid any attention from others. Janarion feels best when he's able to take a break and move physically in some way.

Works Cited

American Psychological Association. (2012, January 1). *Building Your Resilience. American Psychological Association.* Retrieved from https://www.apa.org/topics/resilience

Cleveland Clinic. (2017, December 17). "Anxiety Disorders | Cleveland Clinic." *Cleveland Clinic.* Retrieved from my.clevelandclinic.org/health/diseases/9536-anxiety-disorders

Dijkstra-Kersten, S. M. A., Sitnikova, K., van Marwijk, H. W. J., Gerrits, M. M. J. G., van der Wouden, J. C., Penninx, B. W. J. H. ... Leone, S. S. (2015). Somatisation as a risk factor for incident depression and anxiety. *Journal of Psychosomatic Research, 79*(6), 614–619. Retrieved May 15, 2020. doi: 10.1016/j.jpsychores.2015.07.007

Lieutaud, A., Grenier, K., & Bois, D. (2021). The effects of a mind-body approach, somatic psychoeducation, on anxiety and self-esteem. *Marianne Liebert Inc, 27*(4), 176–186. doi: 10.1089/act.2021.29341.ali.

Maner, J. K., & Schmidt, N. B. (2006). The role of risk avoidance in anxiety. *Behavior Therapy, 37*(2), 181–189.

Mathews, A. (1990). Why worry? The cognitive function of anxiety. *Behaviour Research and Therapy, 28*(6), 455.

Minahan, J., & Rappaport, N. (2012). Anxiety in students a hidden culprit in behavior issues. *Phi Delta Kappan, 94*(4), 34–39.

Pittig, A., Boschet, J. M., Gluck, V. M., & Schneider, K. (2021). Elevated costly avoidance in anxiety disorders: Patients show little downregulation of acquired avoidance in face of competing rewards for approach. *Depression and Anxiety, 38*(3), 361–371.

Rose, J., & Steen, S. (2014). The achieving success everyday group counseling model: Fostering resiliency in middle school students. *Professional School Counseling, 18*(1), 28–37.

Sacco, V. F., & Glackman, W. (1987). Vulnerability, locus of control, and worry about crime. *Canadian Journal of Community Mental Health, 6*(1), 99–111. doi: 10.7870/cjcmh-1987-0007.

Smith Harvey, V. (2007, November). "Resiliency: Strategies for parents and educators." *National Association of School Psychologists (NASP)*. Retrieved May 15, 2022, from www.nasponline.org/publications/periodicals/communique/issues/volume-36-issue-3/resiliency-strategies-for-parents-and-educators

2 What Is Cognitive Behavioral Therapy?

Cognitive behavioral therapy or CBT involves understanding the relationships between thoughts, behaviors, and emotions (Beck & Beck, 2011). CBT considers the person as a whole and integrates strategies to support cognition (thoughts) and behaviors so that overall mood can be beneficially impacted. In addition to considering factors within the person, CBT also incorporates the environment. Although everyone experiences worry, each person has differing resiliency factors. Therefore, the treatment for each child will vary but consideration should be given to temperament, thought patterns, daily life stressors, family support systems, and access to basic needs. Chand, Kuckel, and Huecker (2021) explain this idea with three main areas – underlying beliefs, automatic thoughts, and cognitive distortions:

1 Underlying beliefs – these are the beliefs that have been established throughout our childhood and reinforced by those whom we surround ourselves. These core beliefs are part of what make us who we are and influence our choices and views of the world.

   o An example: the world is full of danger and people who want to hurt me.

2 Automatic thoughts – a thought that occurs reflexively, by habit. Often people with anxiety tend to have more negatively focused automatic thoughts. Take the example of a friend saying, "I can't join you for lunch today."

   o An example: she must be mad at me because I said something I shouldn't have said.

3 Cognitive distortions – ways of thinking that can be rigid and based on a belief rather than truth. These functions can impact actions, thoughts, and feelings. The following are some cognitive distortions often seen with anxiety:

   o All or nothing thinking – thoughts become hung up on one small piece and generalize that statement to everything.

      ▪ An example: I just messed up my painting, I always make mistakes and can't do anything right!

   o Should thinking – where thoughts get stuck on what we should be doing and expectations of ourselves that tend to leave us feeling less than and guilty.

      ▪ An example: I should get all As in my classes and be involved in a lot of extra activities so I can get into a good college.

   o Overgeneralization – thinking gets stuck on one event or thing and large generalizations are made based on that thought. For people who worry, the thinking is often focused on negative generalizations.

      ▪ An example: nobody likes me, they all think I'm weird.

DOI: 10.4324/9781003324782-2

Each of the examples from Chand, Kuckel, and Huecker (2021) explain the more negative and distorted thinking patterns that a person with anxiety may experience. The use of CBT has been found to be beneficial in treating these types of thought patterns (Otte, 2022). Using CBT as a way to support anxiety allows for the opportunity to integrate thoughts, feelings, and actions. For the purposes of this book, we focus on CBT by considering the following as main components in treatment:

- Supporting an awareness of what is occurring across emotions, thoughts, and behaviors.
- Recognizing and then reframing maladaptive thoughts to be more realistic and positive in nature.
- Assessing the situation for what is within our control (our actions) and what is outside of our control (the actions of others).
- Teaching and reinforcing the use of coping strategies that work to calm the mind and body.

Emotions, Thoughts, and Behaviors

Emotions impact thoughts, the physical body, and responses. In someone with anxiety, feelings of worry trigger automatic thoughts that tend to be more distorted, unrealistic, and/or negative in nature. In addition to these automatic thoughts prompted by emotions, behaviors are also stimulated and give rise to physical responses.

Cognitions are influenced by experiences. The thoughts that automatically arise during a challenging situation may be distorted due to past learnings of how situations generally work. For example, if I grew up going to a school where when you look someone in the eye it meant that you wanted to fight, my thoughts would likely jump to "they want to fight me" if I noticed someone looking directly at me.

Behavior responses are impacted by physiology and past learned response patterns. Take the same example of looking someone in the eyes means wanting to fight. When this happens in a situation, the heart will likely begin to race, breathing may increase, and palms may get sweaty as the body prepares to either fight or run away. Behavior includes the actual response to this perceived threat and based on past learnings will likely involve running away from the situation to avoid getting hurt.

Cognitive behavioral therapy includes becoming aware of all of these processes – cognitions, body responses, and actions. This awareness supports an understanding of what is happening within the mind and the body so that automatic thoughts and behaviors can be changed. Understanding emotions, thoughts, and behaviors involves a component of observation and nonjudgement. Practicing non-judgment of emotions is key, as positive emotions like happiness, excitement, joy, and gratitude are often judged as more favorable and preferred. However, we don't only experience positive emotions, we experience all emotions and need a variety of feelings in order to learn and grow. Having the capacity to describe and be aware of all types of emotions while also not judging them has been shown to be related to improved mental health and positive affect (Mandal, Arya, & Pandey, 2012).

Case Studies

Let's consider how emotions may impact the thoughts and behaviors of the four students introduced in Chapter 1.

Braden's Thoughts and Behaviors

Braden is often feeling anxious throughout the day. He feels worried about what types of germs he may come in contact with around the school and stressed when classmates are gone, that he may have or may get whatever they are out sick with that day. When Braden hears a cough, sneeze, or someone blow their nose, his anxiety increases more to fear. When this happens, his body begins to shake, his heart races, and his thoughts begin to spin. Braden considers how he can exit the space and what he needs to do to keep himself healthy. Braden's emotions are largely correlated with his thoughts and behaviors.

- Thoughts: when Braden experiences fear, his mind is overcome with thinking about ways to keep himself safe. Braden worries about the future and the possibility of getting sick which impacts his ability to think clearly. Braden's thoughts include:

  o If I touch any surface that someone else touched, I am going to get sick.
  o There are so many people here, and they could have germs.
  o I just heard someone cough, they must be sick.

- Behavior: Braden's body is under tension so he is more likely to act impulsively (leaving the space) or appear unfocused, darting and moving around the room so that he can avoid germs. Braden's behaviors look like:

  o Unfocused toward others.
  o Difficulty showing expected social behaviors such as looking at someone while they are talking and responding when spoken to.

Mari's Thoughts and Behaviors

Mari's anxiety seems to center around her mom and wanting to make sure that her mom is safe. When Mari is distracted with other tasks and events, her mind is not thinking about her mom. However, as soon as Mari has more down time, her mind begins to wonder about her mom and she feels anxious. When Mari is feeling anxious, her thoughts begin to consider whether something may happen to her mom. She then begins to remember what it was like when her dad died and fears that this will happen to her mom. Mari then begins to think about what it would be like for her if she were left alone without a mom and feels fearful. Mari's thoughts begin to get very negative and focused on her mom dying or getting hurt and then Mari is not able to complete work independently or focus. When her mind thinks this way for too long, she cannot get unstuck unless she talks to her mom and hears that her mom is doing ok. In addition to Mari's thoughts, her body is also under tension. Mari's stomach begins to feel sick, her head hurts, and her shoulders and hands begin to tense.

- Thoughts: when Mari has down time, her thoughts wander more and begin to think about her mom and worry about her mom's safety. Mari goes to the worst-case scenario in her mind and often fears for her mom's safety. Mari's thoughts include:

  o Is mom safe?
  o What if mom isn't safe?
  o Why haven't I heard from mom recently, is she in danger?
  o What will happen if my mom dies too?

- Behaviors: Mari wants her feelings and thoughts to go away. As an attempt to get rid of these thoughts and worries, her behavior is to avoid school work because she is feeling distracted. Mari also works hard to reach out to her mom so that she can validate that her mom is ok so that the unknown can become known again. Mari's behaviors look like:

  o Distracted and not focused on school-related activities
  o Making attempts to find a way to check in on mom

Juliana's Thoughts and Behaviors

Juliana's feelings involve anxiety and anger. These feelings relate to a hyper focus on the issue of concern. It appears that Juliana may become extremely focused on something being a certain way and struggles to think about anything else until she has fixed or completed an action to follow through with the thought of concern.

- Thoughts: when Juliana has high anxiety, her thoughts are focused on a worst-case scenario situation which is often something that is unlikely to happen. Juliana's mind becomes unable to think about anything else, and her thoughts focus on how to stop this feeling and these overpowering thoughts. Juliana's thoughts include:

- ○ This isn't just right like it should be.
- ○ If I don't fix this, it will bother me later and something bad might happen.

- Behaviors: Juliana responds to her thoughts instantly by acting on them by doing something that attempts to fix the feeling of anxiety that she is experiencing. Juliana will react to her thoughts even in the middle of the night when a thought arrives in her head rather than pausing, maybe writing down the plan to wash her clothes as a reminder for tomorrow and returning to bed. Juliana's behaviors look like

- ○ Acting out whatever action will serve to reduce the feeling of anxiety (e.g., fixing the blanket and touching it four times).
- ○ Responding to whatever thoughts come up immediately.

Janarion's Thoughts and Behaviors

Janarion is experiencing somatic symptoms. Somatic symptoms are physical pain that is related to emotions. Janarion experiences stomach pain as well as difficulty in speaking due to increased anxiety. Janarion's feelings relate to being overwhelmed while at school. At school, Janarion feels anxious when there is loud noise as well as when he is around others and there is a potential for him doing something that makes him feel embarrassed. Janarion's thoughts go quickly to the worst that could happen in a situation. Janarion fears that everyone will laugh at him if he says something unexpected. Not only does he worry about this happening, he also worries that once he says something embarrassing, no one will forget he did or said that thing and then will view him as not good enough. Janarion's behaviors serve to protect him by avoiding the situation of going to school at all. Janarion often stays home due to complaints about feeling sick. Janarion's action of avoiding others actually relates to others not seeking out Janarion much which feeds into his thoughts that others don't like him.

- Thoughts: Janarion's thoughts are focused on others' view of him and what he may say or do that could end up causing others to think that he is not good enough for them. Janarion's thoughts include:

- ○ What if I say the wrong thing?
- ○ Everyone will laugh at me and not want to be around me.
- ○ I can't believe I said that. I am so stupid.

- Behaviors: Janarion avoids school and others as a way to impact his emotions and feel calmer as well as to put off thoughts of not being good enough. When Janarion is not able to avoid situations, he doesn't speak as a way to reduce the likelihood of saying something embarrassing. Janarion's behaviors include:

- ○ Avoidance of school and social situations so that he reduces the chance of saying something embarrassing.
- ○ Refusing to talk in social situations to reduce the likelihood of saying something embarrassing.

Reframing Thoughts

When feeling anxious, thoughts tend to focus on the negative and include concerns about what might happen (Chand, Kuckel, & Huecker, 2021). Thoughts that occur while feeling stressed are also not always based in reality (Chand, Kuckel, and Huecker, 2021). Thinking while feeling anxious can be challenging because thoughts can feel out of control and scary. When negative thoughts occur, once consciously recognized, negative thoughts can be challenged and considered in a more realistic way. As the likelihood of the thought happening is considered, thinking may instead be reframed to include the question… what is most likely to happen? Reframing is a way to take back control of negative thoughts and convert them into more positive and supportive thoughts, which ultimately can impact a more positive well-being (Robson & Troutman-Jordan, 2014).

In addition to thinking about "What is most likely to happen" vs. "Worst-case scenario," tasks can be broken down into pieces that feel more attainable as well. When thoughts are acknowledged as inaccurate, there can then be gradual exposure to the stressor. Exposure can occur in multiple ways, by starting with mildly difficult experiences and building to harder experiences (American Psychological Association, 2017). For instance, a person who is terrified of talking to people, especially large groups, can begin by considering one person they feel comfortable talking with as well as a topic that could be comfortable to talk about. Exposure can also include combining relaxation exercises with the fear (American Psychological Association, 2017). The person with anxiety will calm themselves with relaxation exercises and build their capacity to become more comfortable with engaging in their fear. For instance, someone scared of heights will take a deep breath and focus on feeling calm while initially visualizing walking up something tall and then slowly working toward actually walking up something tall.

Case Studies

Braden, Mari, Juliana, and Janarion's thoughts will be examined and reframed. Something to consider is their automatic thoughts are more negative in nature and tend to focus on the worst thing that could possibly happen. Exploring thoughts and feelings involves looking into the thoughts that are occurring and observing what is happening when a stressful event happens and how that is impacting emotions and behaviors. Orson and Larson (2021) found that when thoughts and feelings were encouraged to be explored, student anxiety around completing schoolwork was reduced.

In addition to exploring thoughts, reframing thoughts includes considering what is known about the situation that makes a worst-case scenario unlikely to play out (American Psychological Association, 2022). When reframing thoughts, it is important to remember that although some thoughts can seem quite improbable to someone else, to that person, in that moment, the thought feels very real. Therefore, just saying "that's not true" or "that would never happen" will make the person feel unheard and will not be as helpful as questioning and wondering, "what makes you think that?" or "what data or past experience supports that idea?"

Furthermore, while reframing and exploring thoughts, ideas surrounding exposure will also be considered. Students will gradually dig into components of their anxiety. While doing this, they will build upon their capacity to experience something that makes them feel anxious by identifying a small step they are willing to take to support growth and reduce avoidance.

Exploration of Braden's Thoughts

Braden is often thinking about getting sick. Whenever he is around people, he has thoughts about where their hands have touched, frequently used surfaces, and people's health. All of these observations relate to a fear that people are likely sick and have germs, and their germs will get Braden sick. Braden fears the idea of becoming sick so much that it impacts his daily living and interactions with others. Considering germs is what is always on his mind.

- Core beliefs: Braden sees the world as a dangerous place that can lead to sickness and pain. Braden's beliefs include the idea that if he touches something that is unclean, or if he is around someone who is sick, he will automatically become sick and being sick will be miserable and cause intense pain. Braden also believes that being ill is something to fear and sees illness as threatening to his life.
- Automatic Thoughts:
  - If I touch something another person touches, I will become sick.
  - If I am close to someone with germs, I will become sick.
  - Being around crowds of people leads to illness.
- Cognitive distortions:
  - Everyone I am around has germs which will cause me to be sick.
  - I am unsafe around other people.

- Exploring Thoughts and Feelings (questions for practitioner to ask Braden):

  o What comes up when thinking about going to a large gathering?
  o How do you feel when you think about being around people?
  o What thoughts happen when you are around a lot of people?
  o How can you be around people in a way that feels less uncomfortable?

- Reframing Thoughts: Braden can challenge irrational thoughts by considering:

  o How likely am I to become ill? (I take a lot of precautions by eating healthy, taking care of myself, and taking vitamins)
  o What will happen if I do become ill? (I will likely recover at home but may go to the doctor and get medicine to get better)
  o What am I willing to try to be around people? (I could try being around a small group of people I feel comfortable around and move away if I begin to feel concerned about their health. I can also pay attention to washing my hands and not touching my face which will reduce my chances of getting sick while allowing me to be around others).

Based on Braden's thought patterns, he can gain more control of his thoughts and relief from his anxiety by recognizing thoughts as they occur and evaluating them for their accuracy. When Brayden is able to recognize that his thoughts are negative and, in some way, distorted, he can then challenge them and reframe his thinking, to instead include more action to support regulation of emotions:

- Reframed thought: I feel worried about all of the germs that I may be around. Two things I can do to help myself feel better are: washing my hands and not touching my face. When I begin to feel anxious, I will take five deep breaths to help my body feel more calm and then find someone whom I feel comfortable around.

Exploration of Mari's Thoughts

Mari's thoughts when her mind is not preoccupied center around her mom. Thoughts include where her mom is, what she is doing, whether her mom will make safe choices, if she is safe at that moment, and whether her mom will be able to come home that night. As Mari wonders about her mom, she then begins to think about all of the possibilities of what could be going wrong with her mom. Mari's thoughts often lead to her feeling incredibly anxious and impact her behavior because she is not able to bring her focus back until she knows that her mom is safe.

- Core beliefs: because of Mari's history of her dad dying, she has begun to believe that the world is a dangerous place and that it could take another life of the person she loves. Mari believes that whenever she is not in direct contact with her mom that she must not be safe. Mari fears for her mom's life because she recognizes all of the potential dangers in the world because of experiencing her dad's unexpected death.
- Automatic thoughts:

  o If I can't see, hear, or touch my mom, my mom is unsafe.

- Cognitive distortions:

  o My dad died when I wasn't with him, so this will happen to my mom.
  o The world is unsafe and will take the person I love the most.

- Exploring thoughts and feelings (questions for practitioner to ask Mari):

  o How do you feel when your mom is not close by?
  o What happens that makes you start thinking about your mom?
  o What kind of thoughts arise when you start thinking about mom?
  o What is something that might help you to feel better when you start thinking about your mom?

- Reframing thoughts: Mari can challenge irrational thoughts by considering:

  o What is my mom most likely doing right now? (she's at work)
  o Is this activity generally safe? (yes, my mom sits at a desk)

o Has my mom ever been seriously hurt doing this activity previously? (no she has never been hurt at work before)
o If my mom were hurt, how would that be handled and how would I find out (if mom were hurt she would call the school and your grandparents would then come to let you know that she's hurt and take you to go see her)
o What's something I can do to feel better when I start to worry about mom? (take a break and do something that keeps my mind busy like help a teacher or talk to a friend)

Based on Mari's thought patterns, she can gain comfort and a feeling of calm once she can recognize the negative tendency of her thoughts. The negative thoughts can then be reframed to consider actions that keep her busy. Doing this should support Mari in feeling more relaxed so that she can think more rationally in such a way as:

- Reframed thought: I miss my mom when I am not with her. When I start to miss my mom, I know that having a busy mind helps so I can work on a job or ask to take a break to see someone new. I can remind myself that I will get to see mom later.

Exploration of Juliana's Thoughts

Juliana's thoughts are intense because they take over her mind and impact Juliana so much that she becomes very focused on the thought. When Juliana has these thoughts about something not being quite right or as expected, she feels a need to react to them by following through with an action. Juliana has the expectation that the action will lessen the negative intensity of her thoughts.

- Core beliefs: Juliana has the core belief that she is solely responsible for how things will turn out and therefore, must always be aware of her environment and what needs to be done so that something isn't negatively impacted or something negative doesn't happen. Juliana believes that her actions are directly tied to what will occur next (good or bad). When Juliana has a thought, she believes that she must act on it, or else it will be her fault if something negative happens (e.g., she must pick up the paper that fell on the floor or if someone slips and falls, it will be her fault).
- Automatic thoughts:
  o A dirty dish is seen in the sink when walking out of the house, so Juliana thinks: I need to wash the dishes before I leave even though I'm running late because if I don't ants will get into the house and take over the counter and be impossible to get rid of and none of my friends will want to come over anymore because they will think my house is disgusting.
  o The towel to dry dishes is off center, so Juliana thinks that looks terrible, I must fix it or my mind will think about it all day.
- Exploring thoughts and feelings (questions for practitioner to ask Juliana):
  o How do you feel when something doesn't feel "just right"?
  o What thoughts do you have when you notice something appears not quite as expected?
  o How does it feel to let that thing stay rather than react to the thought that comes up. For example, what would it feel like to not do the dishes when they are dirty?
- Reframing thoughts: Juliana might try to challenge irrational thoughts by considering:
  o What is the worst thing that can happen if I don't act to fix my worry immediately? (The dishes will attract ants that will take over the house and be really hard to get rid of and I won't be able to sleep because I don't want ants near me).
  o How likely is it that this worst thing will actually happen? How do I know? (Unlikely, we rarely have dirty dishes let out for very long)
  o What is most likely to happen? (The dishes will be washed before ants become attracted to them and get in the house).
  o When is a time where I have not acted on my thought, and it turned out ok? (One night I thought I didn't lock the door and decided to stay in bed because I was too cold to get out. I checked the next morning and found that the door was actually locked, and our house was safe).

o   What is something small that I can do to help my worry but doesn't include doing the entire act (e.g., washing the dishes)? (I can put the dishes in the sink and plan to do them when I get home).

Juliana's thoughts involve placing a lot of expectations on herself. Once Juliana is able to examine her beliefs, it would be especially helpful to also evaluate them for the weight that they hold for her to carry (e.g., how much mental space do these worries take up in her mind). It should be brought up that other people can also carry this weight and that sometimes it is best to let thoughts pass without reacting. If Juliana is able to practice some non-reactivity, it can support lessening her anxiety because she will likely recognize that nothing bad will happen when she doesn't act immediately. For example, she can learn that the blanket not being centered on the chair will not cause anything bad to happen.

• Reframed thought: I recognize that this makes me uncomfortable. I am going to try some deep breathing and decide on one small thing I can do that will help me to feel better like put all the dishes in the sink and remind myself that I can do the dishes later.

Exploration of Janarion's Thoughts

Janarion is struggling to connect with his thoughts. Due to Janarion's difficulty in connecting his thoughts and emotions, he is experiencing a lot of physical symptoms. When Janarion is given the skills to feel comfortable in gaining awareness of the emotions that come and go along with his thoughts, his worry will likely relate to a fear of rejection and embarrassment.

• Core beliefs: Janarion has learned that feelings should not be talked about because emotions are private and should be kept to yourself. Janarion feels he is not good enough and that people will not like him even if they know him better. This belief is based on past experiences of others laughing at him and not wanting to play when he was in daycare.
• Automatic thoughts:

  o   When a question is asked, I cannot answer because if I talk, I will say something wrong, be laughed at, and called a loser.
  o   If I say something wrong, everyone will think I'm stupid.
  o   Whenever there's a group of kids close by, there is a high chance if I go up to them I will do something to embarrass myself.

• Exploring thoughts and feelings (questions for practitioner to ask Janarion):

  o   How do you feel when you think about speaking in the classroom?
  o   What thoughts come up when it is your turn to speak?
  o   How would it feel for you to try speaking in front of a couple of other students?
  o   Thinking about talking to peers – who are people you'd be comfortable talking with? What might you feel most comfortable talking about?

• Reframing thoughts: Janarion could challenge these irrational thoughts by asking himself:

  o   What is the worst thing that can happen if I make a mistake? (Everyone will laugh and think I'm not good enough for them)
  o   What will likely happen if I make a mistake (Most people probably won't notice). What if they do notice? How can I help myself to not get stuck in that embarrassment? (I can walk away and try again once I've taken a minute. I can remind myself of mistakes others have made and how easily people forget them.)
  o   What is a small way that I could start to get myself used to talking in public? (I could talk with two friends I feel comfortable around and talk about fishing because we all love fishing).

Janarion's thoughts involve a very negative focus of himself and worry about the perceptions of others. Once Janarion is able to recognize his negative view of himself, it would be helpful if he can look for examples that show positive interactions and his capability to speak with others as a way to build his self-esteem. Janarion can also benefit from making the connection between the physical sensations in his body and the thoughts in his head and emotions he feels. This may help Janarion to better understand the importance of thoughts and emotions and their interrelation with our physical body.

- Reframed thought: it feels scary to be around a lot of other people. I am comfortable with two people in my class and have noticed they seem to like being around me too. I can start by going around just them and relaxing my body by taking a break and breathing when I notice I'm getting worried.

As this practice on reframing thinking has shown, thoughts can be re-worked and within our control. However, when it comes to anxiety, there are still other aspects wrapped up in situations of worry that are outside of our control. Helping to support students in recognizing what is within their control and what is outside of their control can be empowering to help in considering what they have authority over and then letting go of that of which there is nothing that they can do.

What Is Within Our Control and What Is Out of Our Control?

A ball comes flying in the air and hits you in the head. Is it your fault? Well, it depends on how you think about the situation. Let's consider what is within your control first. There is always the option to be extra aware of your surroundings, and then move when you see a ball come flying at you. You have control of yourself and your choices. What you do not have control over is the ball and any intent behind the ball. No matter how aware you are of your environment, that ball still could hit you. The ball may be flying faster than you can move, the ball may be out of your eyesight, or the ball may catch a gust of wind and move with you as you move. When thinking about situations in this way, we remember that oftentimes there are pieces of the problem that are within our control, like how we choose to respond, cope, or fix the situation. We also recognize that there are parts of a problem that are outside of our control, including other people's actions, the environment, and certain schedules. Some parts of life are more fixed and solid and outside of our control, while other pieces are more flexible and moldable, and something that we can work to change or influence.

Anxiety has been found to increase when perception of control is reduced (Hofmann, 2005). In addition, lack of control has also been found to impact performance (Walker & Nordin-Bates, 2010). Based on these findings, those with anxiety can especially benefit from evaluating a situation and considering what they have control over in that situation, and how they may influence a response. In turn, what is outside of their control should be acknowledged and limits accepted. Mental capacity can then instead focus on what is able to be changed.

Case Studies

Considering each of the four students, we will walk through what is within their control and what is outside of their control and can be let go of.

Braden and Control

Braden's worry about germs impacts his own actions and thoughts. However, Braden also has considered what is happening outside of himself such as other people's actions and cleanliness of events. Braden has control of himself, but limited control over what is happening around him and even his true likelihood to become sick.

- Within Braden's control:
  - o Washing hands.
  - o Limiting touch of highly used surfaces.
  - o Limiting being around large crowds of people.
- Outside of Braden's control:
  - o Whether people with an illness are around him.
  - o Precautions that others take with their cleanliness practices.
  - o Whether he ends up getting sick.

Mari and Control

Mari's thoughts related to her mom include notions of worries that are largely outside of her control, including her mom's actions and whereabouts. Although Mari may feel that she has little control over this worry, there are pieces that she has control over. Mari has control over her recognition of her own thoughts and how much her thoughts spiral.

- Within Mari's control:
    - Recognizing thoughts.
    - Reminding herself that her mom is likely safe by remembering where her mom is and the risk associated with that place and activity.
    - Continuing or starting an activity that serves as a distractor.
- Outside of Mari's control:
    - Whether her mother is safe.
    - Where her mom is currently located.
    - What her mom is doing.

Juliana and Control

Juliana has the belief that she holds more control than she does in situations. Juliana feels that her actions can reduce the likelihood of bad things happening, and that by continuing to act on her thoughts, her mind will feel more at ease. The more that Juliana continues to act on her thoughts, the less she is able to feel settled with the idea of something unexpected happening.

- Within Juliana's control:
    - Recognizing her thoughts and choosing not to act on them.
- Outside of Juliana's control:
    - Other people's actions and behavior.
    - Generally, whether something unwanted will happen.

Janarion and Control

Janarion is placing much of the control of stress and fear onto himself. Janarion is assuming that by not participating in discussions or activities, he then does not need to be concerned about the risk for what others say. Janarion does not have the capacity to determine what others say, even if he alters his actions in an effort to do so.

- Within Janarion's control:
    - How he responds to others' negative or positive comments.
    - Who he chooses to spend his time around.
    - What he says or does when around peers.
- Outside of Janarion's control:
    - How others respond to Janarion.
    - Type of comments that are made to Janarion (negative or positive).

Considering each student's worries in this way helps to point out the importance of recognizing thoughts as a way to also gain control and understanding. People can be mean, disappointing, unexpected, and surprising. We can understand and accept those pieces of others but cannot change them. What we can change is our response (e.g., leaving the room when someone says something unkind). We can also change our thought (e.g., I am scared something bad will happen but know that is unlikely). Although control is lacking in some aspects of anxiety, coping strategies can be used as a method to reduce the feeling of worry related to the unexpected and unknown.

Coping Strategies

Coping includes thoughts and behavior responses to both internal and external situations that have been identified as stressful (Taylor & Stanton, 2007). Coping can come in many different forms but has the goal of reducing tension within the mind and the body when intense emotions are felt. In their 2008 article, *Coping with Stress*, Bartram and Gardner describe coping as being broken into two focuses:

1 Problem-focused coping:

  o Create a plan of action.
  o Try to see something from another perspective.
  o Ask for help.
  o Apply time-management skills.
  o Be assertive.
  o Consider past experiences.

2 Emotion-focused coping:

  o Confide in someone else.
  o Engage in physical exercise.
  o Write down thoughts and feelings.
  o Distract attention by working on something else.
  o Spend time with pets.
  o Practice relaxation or meditation.
  o Challenge negative thoughts.

Bartram and Gardner (2008) further explain that when a situation feels more unchangeable and outside of the person's control, emotion-focused coping is most beneficial; and when a situation is changeable and within the person's control, problem-focused coping is a better fit. In addition to considering emotion- and problem-focused coping strategies, Taylor and Stanton (2007) identified that coping strategies that focus on action, optimism, personal control, and positive sense of self can improve coping long-term. The way in which a person copes is unique to them but should also be something that is a positive outlet, related to what they need, and not likely to harm the person further in some way. For instance, maladaptive coping strategies such as cutting can cause relief in the short term but in the long term lead to more psychological and physical safety concerns (Bartram & Gardner, 2008). Therefore, when considering how to support students with anxiety, strategies should involve efforts to enhance the student's capacity to positively help themselves.

Case Studies

We'll now consider what sort of coping strategies may be most beneficial to Braden, Mari, Juliana, and Janarion's situations.

Braden's Coping Strategies

Much of Braden's anxiety involves pieces outside of his control, therefore emotion-focused coping strategies will be most supportive for Braden. Braden has shared that something that really helps to keep his mind feeling calm is reading a story or writing. Braden enjoys fiction stories about superheroes and has been working on his own novel.

• Coping Option 1: reading as a distraction and re-set when Braden recognizes he's starting to feel upset and struggling to think logically.
• Coping Option 2: journaling as a way for Braden to get his feelings onto paper, and then challenging the thoughts that arise that appear to be cognitive distortions.

- Coping Option 3: talking through worries with someone he identifies as supportive in a way that identifies the thoughts that come up for him, and walking through the distorted thinking to get to a reframed thought.

It is really important for Braden to continually practice reframing his thoughts so that he can begin to reframe negative thoughts into more accurate/positive thoughts automatically. By practicing this response in multiple formats (e.g., writing and talking), Braden will likely become more skilled at doing this independently.

Mari's Coping Strategies

Much of Mari's anxiety relates to occurrences outside of her control as it surrounds what her mom is doing. Therefore, emotion-focused coping can be most helpful for Mari. Mari feels calm once she is able to talk with someone. Talking with an adult helps Mari to become aware of her thoughts and the unlikelihood of them happening, while focusing on what is most likely to occur (e.g., mom is safe and at work). Talking through her thoughts and recognizing their pattern with an adult helps Mari to feel safe and calm. Pairing this with movement is also supportive for Mari as physically doing something seems to help to re-set her thinking and helps her body to feel calmer.

- Coping Option 1: going to see a supportive adult when Mari recognizes the first signs of anxiety (by paying attention to her body and thoughts). This adult can support in bringing her back to a state of calm by doing something together in a relaxing space or going for a walk.
- Coping Option 2: walking with a supportive adult while talking through her thoughts and feelings. This discussion should include considering what is within her control (what she is doing) and what is outside of her control (what mom is doing).
- Coping Option 3: first talking through feelings with a supportive adult and identifying what is most likely occurring, and the cognitive distortions that are happening in her thoughts. Then playing a physical game such as basketball.

With Mari's body responding best to movement, practicing reframing her thoughts and considering control while moving may support her body in getting the physical release that it craves. Even if the discussion occurs separately and Mari is then allowed to do something active before or after the discussion, she may feel better because she tends to hold onto a lot of her stress in her body. Moving is a way in which she can release the tension.

Juliana's Coping Strategies

Juliana's anxiety is largely surrounding pieces that are within her control, and therefore problem-focused coping will be most impactful. Her thoughts are frequently shifting from one thing to the next, and she feels compelled to act on stressful thoughts that arise. What appears to be most beneficial to Juliana is using a decision-making process to consider whether there needs to be an action immediately or if the action can wait or doesn't need to occur. Juliana can be supported by getting help in talking through problem-solving with someone else to reinforce expected actions and talk about anxious thoughts that arise.

- Coping Option 1: creating a decision-making model and reviewing potential options before automatically jumping into action when a thought arises.
- Coping Option 2: reframing thoughts by considering what is most likely to happen if she does not act on a thought.
- Coping Option 3: check-ins with a supportive adult to support expected decision-making and reinforce accountability.

Juliana tends to get stuck in her thoughts and allows them to control a lot of her actions. When Juliana is able to teach her mind to slow down and evaluate her decisions, she can become less reactive and more accepting of the moment.

Janarion's Coping Strategies

Much of Janarion's anxiety is within his control as it involves his own responses toward others. However, there are also pieces of his worry that are outside of his control, like how other people will respond. When Janarion recognizes that his body is beginning to hold onto stress and worry by becoming physically ill, it is important that he work to re-set his body by physically moving. For Janarion, the physical act of movement can help him in releasing stress and support him in feeling calmer.

- Coping Option 1: having a pre-planned break option that might include:
  - A walking route.
  - An obstacle course with pre-planned movement exercises (e.g., throw the medicine ball ten times, do five pushups, do ten jumping jacks, and jump on 1 foot for 30 seconds).
  - Going to another room to do a job for someone.
- Coping Option 2: evaluating the situation and considering what is most likely to happen versus what is the worst-case scenario (reflect upon positive past experiences).
- Coping Option 3: creating a plan with a trusted adult to build upon social interactions and gain confidence.

Janarion is very stuck in believing he is not good enough and that others will feel this way about him too. Therefore, it is important to support Janarion in thinking through how he might interact with others and consider what is most likely to happen versus what is the worst-case scenario. In addition, because movement is identified as a supportive option for Janarion, he can be sure to incorporate that as a way to support his body in feeling more calm.

When determining a coping plan that can be helpful, the student should always be a part of this discussion. It is important that the discussion also involves not just what may be something the student likes to do but also something that helps their mind and body to feel calm. For instance, even though a student enjoys walking around the school, if this does not support them in re-starting their brain and helping their body to feel more calm, it's not a great coping strategy to continue using. In addition, the students' coping plan should also include ideas on how to build upon skills to support optimism, personal control, and self-love (Taylor & Stanton, 2007) while giving consideration to whether it should be emotionally focused or problem focused (Bartram & Gardner, 2008).

CBT Conclusion

When utilizing CBT as a therapeutic approach, individuals are encouraged to recognize their thoughts and pay attention to how some thoughts may be negative in nature and come on automatically. Becoming more aware of thoughts helps to break this cycle of negative thinking and promote more realistic and positive thinking. In addition, CBT acknowledges that thoughts, feelings, and behaviors are all connected. When thoughts change, emotions and behaviors are also impacted. Therefore, coping strategies should be thoughtfully considered as to what will work best with the amount of control the student has in the situation, what opportunities can build skills, and how to promote self-love and personal control.

Works Cited

American Psychological Association Division 12. (2017, July). *What Is Exposure Therapy?*

American Psychological Association. (2022). *Handout 27: 5 Steps of Cognitive Restructuring Instructions.* Retrieved from www.apa.org/pubs/books/supplemental/Treatment-for-Postdisaster-Distress/Handout-27.pdf.

Bartram, D., & Gardner, D. (2008). Coping with stress. *In Practice, 30*(4), 228–231.

Beck, J. S., & Beck, A. T. (2011). *Cognitive behavior therapy.* New York: Basics and beyond. Guilford Publication.

Chand, S. P., Kuckel, D. P., & Huecker, M. R. (2021). Cognitive behavior therapy. In *StatPearls [Internet].* StatPearls Publishing.

Hofmann, S. G. (2005). Perception of control over anxiety mediates the relation between catastrophic thinking and social anxiety in social phobia. *Behaviour Research and Therapy, 43*(7), 885–895.

Mandal, S. P., Arya, Y. K., & Pandey, R. (2012). Mental health and mindfulness: Mediational role of positive and negative affect. *SIS Journal of Projective Psychology and Mental Health, 19*(2), 150–159.

Orson, C. N., & Larson, R. W. (2021). Helping teens overcome anxiety episodes in project work: The power of reframing. *Journal of Adolescent Research,* 36(2), 127–153.

Otte, C. (2022). Cognitive behavioral therapy in anxiety disorders: Current state of the evidence. *Dialogues in Clinical Neuroscience, 13*(4), 413–421. doi: 10.31887/DCNS.2011.13.4/cotte.

Robson, J. P. Jr, & Troutman-Jordan, M. (2014). A concept analysis of cognitive reframing. *Journal of Theory Construction & Testing, 18*(2), 55–59.

Taylor, S. E., & Stanton, A. L. (2007). Coping resources, coping processes, and mental health. *Annual Review of Clinical Psychology, 3*, 377–401.

Walker, I. J., & Nordin-Bates, S. M. (2010). Performance anxiety experiences of professional ballet dancers the importance of control. *Journal of Dance Medicine & Science, 14*(4), 133–145.

3 How Can Mindfulness Support CBT?

What Is Mindfulness?

Mindfulness involves being in a state of awareness and acceptance without judgment or reactivity while also maintaining attention to the current moment (Bishop et al., 2004). A person who practices mindfulness does not necessarily have less invasive thoughts but is at ease with the thoughts that do arise (Teper, Segal, & Inzlicht, 2013). Mindfulness practice brings the mind back to the moment whenever it begins to wander. Thoughts are acknowledged but allowed to float past.

Mindfulness has been described as a practice that supports overall focused attention by helping the mind to see things more clearly (Greenland, 2015). Mindfulness is beneficial to all and supports well-being, reduced negative emotions, and lessened anxiety (Weare, 2013). Its definition and benefits can be described to children and adolescents in the following ways:

- Mindfulness helps to teach the brain to be in the moment and not think about something that has happened in the past or is about to happen.
  - Example for practitioner to state to child or adolescent:
    - Have you ever felt like you can't sleep because your mind just won't stop thinking about things?
      - Whenever that happens, your mind is struggling to be in the present moment and that can cause worry and make it hard to relax and fall asleep. Starting a mindfulness practice that brings the mind back to the moment can help to calm the brain. Such a practice might look like focusing on the breath and counting. For example, breathe in and count 1…2…3… hold the breath and count 2…2…3… and let the breath out for 3…2…3… and continue doing this while focusing on counting and the breath.
- Mindfulness can support awareness of actions within the moment.
  - Example for practitioner to state to child or adolescent:
    - Have you ever experienced finishing a bag of chips and being surprised that they were all gone?
      - Being mindful of what you're eating helps you to savor each chip and be aware of when you truly feel full.
- Mindfulness helps the mind to be present in fun activities which can lead to experiencing more positive emotions.
  - Example for practitioner to state to child or adolescent:
    - Have you ever left a day of fun you've been looking forward to for a while and recognized that the day passed so quickly you didn't take in all of the excitement?
      - Being mindful while experiencing fun supports your mind in being present of all that is happening including the sounds, sights, tastes, and smells.

DOI: 10.4324/9781003324782-3

How to Cultivate Mindfulness

A regular practice of mindfulness can support more awareness in the moment along with acceptance of whatever emotions arise (Teper, Segal, & Inzlicht, 2013). The more the mind continues to come back to the moment, the better able it is to do this automatically. When the mind is aware of wandering, that in and of itself is mindfulness. Children and adolescents tend to understand the benefits of practicing mindfulness soon after being introduced to the practice and may reflect with such statements as, "my body feels more calm," "I feel really good," or "that helped my body to feel lighter." Mindfulness can be cultivated in many different ways. People tend to work to cultivate mindfulness through a focus on breath work, movement, creativity, or visualization.

Breath Work

Breathing is something that we do all the time. However, when utilizing breath work, mindful meditation is one way to become more aware of the physical act of breathing and the thoughts that are present within the mind. When focusing on breath as a meditative practice, attention is paid to the awareness of breathing in and out. Formal practices (structured meditation practice where time is devoted specifically to meditation) and informal practices (bringing attention back to the moment and breath in everyday life) have been found to relate to a feeling of calm and balance (Juneau, Shankland, & Dambrun, 2020). There are many options for pre-recorded and streamed meditation practices including the use of websites, apps, and podcasts. A mindfulness practice can be mostly quiet where the focus is on breathing in…. and out…., or a practice may be more specific and focus on a consideration of generosity, letting go, or sharing love.

Movement

Moving with mindfulness is believed to enhance social connections, relationships, and overall mood (Lucas, Klepin, Porges, & Rejeski, 2018). Whenever movement is included with mindfulness, attention is related to how the body feels within space, and breath is coordinated with movement. Mindfulness is often associated with slow and steady movements like yoga, but mindfulness can be paired with most any type of movement. The focus when pairing movement with breath and in-the-moment thinking is that our mind needs to continue to be brought back to the present. This can be done by noticing how the body is moving, what thoughts arise within the mind, how breathing feels, and what sounds are noticed.

Creativity

Being creative in a mindful way can simply include observing and noticing all of the parts involved in creation. The creative project may have a purpose such as building a sculpture, designing a room, or creating a photo album. Creativity can also be about what is occurring in the moment without a distinct purpose – coloring, free drawing, or writing whatever comes to mind. The important piece with creativity and mindfulness is that there is concentration and awareness around what is happening within the body and the mind while creating. There may be more attention to how the pen feels in the hand, color selections, which way the pencil moves, or how the hand leans against the paper. Being creative while being mindful is less about the product and more about the process and noticing each step along the way.

Visualization

Visualization practices involve focusing on something specific. It is like having a movie described out loud while the picture is created within the mind with your eyes closed. Visualization allows for the practice of controlling thoughts and working through moments when your mind may want to wander. Visualization may include reminiscing on a favorite memory, being very aware of all the colors from a past event, or thinking about a future goal. The visualization can be led in person, or it might be something that is listened to from a pre-recorded session through an app, Cd, podcast, or website.

Informal Practice

In addition to these more formal, structured practices, mindfulness can be practiced informally in everyday situations. Whenever a person notices thoughts that come up that aren't related to the present, that is practicing mindfulness. Mindfulness in everyday life may look like paying close attention to all that occurs within the body when doing an activity such as tennis, walking, or swimming. Mindfulness can also include becoming aware of all the steps involved in daily tasks like brushing your teeth or showering. In addition, mindfulness can be cultivated by taking in the world and noticing sounds, paying attention to the colors, and feeling the air on your skin.

Mindfulness Practices for Students

Each of these practices for mindfulness can be utilized for children and adolescents with anxiety. The beauty of mindfulness is its versatility. Mindfulness allows for opportunities to be used daily to support general feelings of calm and is also able to support in regulating intense emotions. Mindfulness can be introduced and normalized by observing adults modeling their own practice as well as being offered opportunities to practice mindfulness as a whole group with peers.

Emotion Awareness

A benefit that mindfulness has shown is an increased awareness and acceptance of emotions (Gratz & Tull, 2010). Oftentimes, people with anxiety attempt to avoid certain feelings and may have a difficult time accepting emotions that arise. However, practicing mindfulness can be beneficial because it allows for the awareness that all emotions come and go. Emotions are not permanent and recognizing this through mindfulness practices can promote further acceptance of all emotions whether they are positive or negative, and support in regulating emotions (Gratz & Tull, 2010). Mindfulness is a reminder that just as clouds float in and out, emotions too come and go but don't stay forever. Having a willingness to acknowledge emotions and become aware of their impact on behavior and thoughts is supportive in preparing the mind to be ready to consider how negative automatic thoughts and judgments can be reframed through cognitive behavioral therapy (CBT) techniques.

Mindfulness and CBT

Mindfulness can be cultivated in many different ways. Pairing mindfulness with CBT offers an opportunity to pay attention in the moment while considering what is most needed in order to support more positive thoughts, feelings, and behavior. As Baer and Sauer (2009) point out, mindfulness and CBT have similarities as well as differences in their approaches which allow for the opportunity to offer an integrative approach that utilizes the strengths of each to support emotion regulation. A similarity of mindfulness and CBT includes an awareness of thoughts and the impact of thoughts and feelings on the body. A difference between the two therapies is that mindfulness tends to focus on being aware and accepting of thoughts and emotions that arise without reacting to or judging them, while CBT has a focus on reframing thoughts. Research has found mindfulness-based interventions (MBIs) and CBT to perform similarly in the support of anxiety (Hofmann & Gomez, 2017). Mindfulness and CBT both have something to offer for students with anxiety, which is why both approaches are utilized throughout the sessions in this book.

CBT approach:

- A focus on the relation between thoughts, feelings, and behaviors.
- Analysis of thoughts in reframing thoughts.
- Practice in reframing thoughts.
- Consideration of environmental factors that impact behavior and thoughts.

Mindfulness:

- Observing and accepting emotions and thoughts that arise.
- Not judging or reacting to emotions or thoughts and recognizing that they will come and go and are not permanent.
- Practice in bringing the mind to the current moment.

Case Studies

Let's look at each of our students and explore how CBT and mindfulness together can support anxiety.

Braden – CBT and Mindfulness

CBT – analyzing thoughts: Braden's thoughts are stuck in a loop of negative thinking. When he is in situations that are less controlled (e.g., lots of people, new and different environment), his thoughts begin to jump to a worry of coming into contact with germs and then getting sick. Braden works to control these thoughts as a way to reduce his worries. However, this automatic reaction to thoughts ends up reinforcing their existence and then he avoids situations he finds challenging.

- Automatic thoughts:
  - If I touch something another person touches, I will become sick.
  - If I am close to someone with germs, I will become sick.
  - Being around crowds of people leads to illness.
- Cognitive distortions:
  - Everyone who I am around has germs that will cause me to be sick.
  - I am unsafe around other people.

Mindfulness – acceptance of thoughts and emotions: Braden can utilize mindfulness as a way to become aware of when his thoughts begin to jump from the present moment. Braden can do this by becoming aware of when he begins to make judgments about the current situation or attempt to predict what will happen. By bringing his thoughts back to the current moment, Braden is reminded of what he knows to be true at that time. He can be comforted by the fact that he likely feels healthy and safe at that moment, and if he does not, recognizing that all feelings are ok and pass. Mindfulness can support Braden to lean into challenging emotions by recognizing what thoughts, feelings, and body sensations arise within each moment (Hayes, 2022).

CBT – reframing thoughts: once Braden is aware of his thoughts and considers his safety within the current moment, he is able to reframe thoughts to be more accurate:

- Reframed thought: I feel worried about all of the germs that I may be around. Two things I can do to help myself feel better are: washing my hands and not touching my face. When I begin to feel anxious, I will take five deep breaths to help my body feel more calm and then find someone whom I feel comfortable around.

Mindfulness – practice: a mindful/meditative strategy that Braden may use at that moment is 5-4-3-2-1 grounding technique discussed later in this book and found with Appendix F-A. This technique can be useful for him because it helps him to find concrete things in the room that he can focus on and then supports him with existing within the moment.

Mari – CBT and Mindfulness

CBT – analyzing thoughts: Mari's thoughts jump to her mom whenever she is not with her. Once this happens, Mari's thoughts run wild and begin to make up their own reality that causes stress and worry for Mari about her mom's safety.

- Automatic thoughts:

  o If I can't see, hear, or touch my mom, that means my mom is unsafe.

- Cognitive distortions:

  o My dad died when I wasn't with him, so this will happen to my mom.
  o The world is unsafe and will take the person I love the most.

Mindfulness – acceptance of thoughts and emotions: grounding in breath can support Mari whenever she notices intrusive thoughts arising. Mari can gain skill to acknowledge these thoughts but not react physically (e.g., dialing mom's number) or with thought (e.g., continuing to analyze and consider what negative thing may have happened to mom). The more that Mari is able to practice and talk through this way of thinking, the more she can recognize that these thoughts will come and go and do not directly tie to an outcome. This awareness can support Mari in resisting the automatic notion that has occurred in the past where she then begins to fear for her mom and consider all of the worst-case scenarios that could be happening at that moment. Then instead, Mari can acknowledge her fear and sit with that feeling, knowing that it will pass and she does not need to act.

CBT – reframing thoughts: by bringing her thoughts back to the moment, Mari can be more open to considering what is most likely occurring for her mom and recognize the distortion in her thinking.

- Reframed thought: I miss my mom when I am not with her. When I start to miss my mom I know that having a busy mind helps so I can work on a job or ask to take a break to see someone new. I can remind myself that I will get to see mom later.

Mindfulness – practice: considering a more mindful approach, Mari might be able to bring her mind back to the current moment first by introducing some sort of creative activity. When Mari switches from what she was doing to work on being creative, she has the chance to re-focus her brain on the activity at hand and recognize all of the opportunities with the project to be conscious of that moment. Before completing the creativity project, Mari can be reminded of the importance of grounding herself with her breath.

Juliana – CBT and Mindfulness

CBT – analyzing thoughts: Juliana sees the world with specific expectations. When something in her environment does not match that expectation, Juliana's mind gets stuck and feels an impulse to react or judge and somehow "fix" whatever is not at her expectation.

- Automatic thoughts:
  o A dirty dish is seen in the sink when walking out of the house, I need to wash the dishes before I leave even though I'm running late because if I don't ants will get into the house and take over the counter and be impossible to get rid of and none of my friends will want to come over anymore because they will think my house is disgusting.
  o Something is not perfect, I must fix it or it will cause problems.
- Exploring thoughts and feelings (questions for practitioner to ask the student):
  o How do you feel when something doesn't feel "just right"?
  o What thoughts do you have when you notice something appears not quite as expected?
  o How does it feel to let that thing stay rather than react to the thought that comes up (e.g., what would it feel like to not do the dishes?)

Mindfulness – acceptance of thoughts and emotions: mindfulness will support Juliana in being able to practice bringing her attention to her thoughts and emotions. As Juliana recognizes the power of these thoughts and ties her thoughts to the emotions she is feeling, she may notice certain thoughts or events trigger certain emotions. With her awareness, as Juliana becomes better able to sit with her thoughts and feelings and learns that nothing bad will happen if she doesn't react, she may then be able to more easily lean into feelings she may have previously judged as negative.

CBT – reframing thoughts: through Juliana recognizing how much power her thoughts have over her actions, she can then work to take that power back through reframing her thoughts into more realistic scenarios.

- Reframed thought: I recognize that this makes me uncomfortable. I am going to try some deep breathing and decide on one small thing I can do that will help me to feel better like put all the dishes in the sink and remind myself that I can do the dishes later.

Mindfulness – practice: introducing Juliana to mindfulness and supporting her in its practice of guided breath awareness and visualization would allow Juliana practice opportunities to recognize when her thoughts are straying from the moment and moving toward a judgment or reactive state of mind. Supporting Juliana in thinking in this way may reduce her impulsive actions as well as her thoughts around control and feelings of being anxious.

Juliana would do well with setting up a regular guided mindfulness practice. She might try multiple modalities of mindful listening to help her determine what she views as most beneficial and favorable for her. Guided meditation options should include: mindful meditation with a focus on breath awareness, visualization practices, or movement paired with awareness of breath and body.

Janarion – CBT and Mindfulness

CBT – analyzing thoughts: Janarion struggles to be aware and accepting of his thoughts and emotions that arise. Janarion judges unexpected feelings (e.g., sad, mad, frustrated, hurt, etc.) as bad and then attempts to change those feelings through distraction or avoidance.

- Automatic thoughts:
  - A question is asked. I cannot answer because if I talk, I will say something wrong, be laughed at, and called a loser.
  - If I say something wrong, everyone will think I'm stupid.
  - Social situations are chances for me to be embarrassed.

- Exploring thoughts and feelings (questions for practitioner to ask the student):
  - How do you feel when you think about speaking in the classroom?
  - What thoughts come up when it is your turn to speak?
  - How would it feel for you to try speaking in front of a couple of other students?

Mindfulness – acceptance of thoughts and emotions: Janarion could benefit from practicing mindfulness as a way to recognize and observe his thoughts and emotions as they arise. Without reacting, and simply just noticing his thoughts, Janarion may recognize that certain thoughts feel more negative and when these thoughts arise, his emotions feel more negative also. This recognition may help Janarion to break out of irrational thought patterns and notice that thoughts and emotions are not permanent and can be supported simply through an awareness of what is happening within the mind and the body.

CBT – reframing thoughts: once Janarion is able to practice not reacting to his thoughts, he may be more aware of the potential benefits participating in a conversation can bring (e.g.; more friendships).

- Reframed thought: it feels scary to be around a lot of other people. I am comfortable with two people in my class and have noticed they seem to like being around me too. I can start by going around just them and relaxing my body by taking a break and breathing when I notice I'm getting worried.

Mindfulness – practice: for Janarion, he may most benefit from a mindfulness practice where there is another person whom he can talk to throughout the process. This other person could offer Janarion an opportunity to listen to how they acknowledge, accept, and observe their own thoughts. A mindfulness practice that may support Janarion is walking or moving while practicing, observing, and accepting thoughts and emotions that arise. Janarion may also benefit from some guided movement practices where he listens to a mindfulness practice that walks through each of the movements involved in the physical activity and incorporates this movement with breath (e.g., mindful walking).

Works Cited

Baer, R. A., & Sauer, S. (2009). Mindfulness and cognitive behavioral therapy: A commentary on Harrington and Pickles. *Journal of Cognitive Psychotherapy, 23*(4), 324–332.

Bishop, S. R., Lau, M., Shapiro, S., Carlson, L., Anderson, N. D., Carmody, J. ... Devins, G. (2004). Mindfulness: A proposed operational definition. *Clinical Psychology: Science and Practice, 11*(3), 230–241.

Gratz, K. L., & Tull, M. T. (2010). Emotion regulation as a mechanism of change in acceptance-and mindfulness-based treatments. *Assessing Mindfulness and Acceptance Processes in Clients: Illuminating the Theory and Practice of Change, 2,* 107–133.

Greenland, S. K. (2015). *Teaching mindfulness skills to kids and teens.* Chapter 21: Neurobiological Modeles of Meditation Practices: Implications for Applications with Youth. P. 402–426. Guilford Publications.

Hayes, S. (2022, August 13). *The most important skill set in Mental Health.* Steven C. Hayes, PhD. Retrieved August 16, 2022 https://stevenchayes.com/the-most-important-skill-set-in-mental-health/?fbclid=IwAR0m-Ly7910hcC5H4iei9o5FjvW7pDpcBoZYbd8RNzHuHUlaIAW4i82YpKBU

Hofmann, S. G., & Gómez, A. F. (2017, September 18). Mindfulness-based interventions for anxiety and depression. *Psychiatr Clin North Am, 40*(4), 739–749. doi: 10.1016/j.psc.2017.08.008.

Juneau, C., Shankland, R., & Dambrun, M. (2020). Trait and state equanimity: The effect of mindfulness-based meditation practice. *Mindfulness, 11*(7), 1802–1812.

Lucas, A. R., Klepin, H. D., Porges, S. W., & Rejeski, W. J. (2018). Mindfulness-based movement: A polyvagal perspective. *Integrative Cancer Therapies, 17*(1), 5–15.

Teper, R., Segal, Z. V., & Inzlicht, M. (2013). Inside the mindful mind: How mindfulness enhances emotion regulation through improvements in executive control. *Current Directions in Psychological Science, 22*(6), 449–454.

Weare, K. (2013, April). *Evidence for the Impact of Mindfulness on Children and Young People.* Mood Disorders Centre.

4   How to Use this Book

Student Selection

This book is intended for use with students that struggle with anxiety. Sessions can be completed one on one or with a small group of students. It is recommended that there are not more than five students in the small group so that there is an opportunity for all students in the group to share and so that students feel comfortable in sharing with those around them. When the group size goes up, response time is more limited, and students tend to be more cautious of what they are sharing and may be less open about their true concerns.

Students should be close in age if they are part of the group but could be across grades (e.g., fourth and fifth graders may pair well in a group but fourth and sixth graders would not pair as well). In addition to thinking about the size and age of the group, the dynamics of personalities should also be considered. Thoughtful conversations with teachers about who may fit best together will likely support the creation of a group that is beneficial to all involved.

Students selected to work through the nine sessions might have a diagnosis related to anxiety, including generalized anxiety, a specific phobia, social anxiety, or panic disorder. Some students may not have a diagnosis but struggle with worrying, and their worry impacts their functioning at school or at home. When determining if a student would be a good fit in the program, it can be useful to explain a general overview to guardians or teachers with the following language:

> The program includes nine-week sessions where your student and I meet one time per week for thirty minutes. During the time together, we will be working to build a relationship so that it feels comfortable for them to explore their emotions and discuss their worry. Strategies will be shared that include reframing of negative thoughts as well as calm coping techniques such as mindfulness. Each week a summary of learning together will be shared out with you. Weekly updates will also include ideas for continued learning in the classroom and at home.

Once determining fit and whether sessions will be completed one on one or in a small group, send home the permission form for a guardian to complete (Appendix A) and have guardians complete the feedback form (Appendix B-G) and the student's teacher complete the teacher feedback form (Appendix B-T). Once all materials have been returned, begin working through Chapters 5 through 13.

Strategies Utilized in Chapters 5–15

Throughout Chapters 5–15, strategies are included that are in line with cognitive behavioral therapy (CBT) and mindfulness-based practices and are not of original creation. For instance, the variety of breathing techniques offered in each chapter have been utilized to calm the body by many cultures across the world. In addition, the environment and conversation suggestions are pieces that have been found to support emotion regulation within the school and home setting but were not created

DOI: 10.4324/9781003324782-4

by this author (e.g., a calm space, worry box, family-guided conversations). Credit is given, when the origination of the idea was able to be identified.

Chapters 5–13 Explained

The following nine chapters (Chapters 5–13) are meant to be utilized by school-based clinicians for use with students who struggle with anxiety. This book focuses on students that are in fourth through eighth grade. However, the sessions do provide adaptations to consider for younger and older students. Each chapter includes three main sections: the outline, clinician notes, and teacher and guardian summary/homework.

Outline:

- The outline is intended to be a quick reference option that is straight to the point for a busy clinician. Although preparation can help the session to run smoothly, the outline provides the option for the clinician to easily reference what can be said and done in a short and succinct format. Note that the essential speaking text is differentiated by the color blue. In each outline, there is included:
    - Focus – The goal of this chapter is outlined.
    - Learning targets – Expectations of what the students will be able to do after completing the session are described.
    - Materials needed – a bulleted list of all of the pintables needed for the session in addition to any supplemental materials.
    - Introduction/assessment – this section focuses on checking in with the student, gathering data with assessments, and discussing any homework assigned from the last meeting. Checking in with the student happens as a way to build the relationship and allow an opening for any concerns that may be on the student's mind. Assessments are completed so that progress can be monitored and changes can be made as needed to better support the student in areas in which they continue to struggle. The homework check-in shows the student that whatever homework was given to them will be followed up on and helps them to be accountable to their growth while not in session.
    - Main lesson – focus on new learning and creating an opportunity to practice and reflect together.
    - Wrap-up – summary of the time together is given to the student along with expectations of what to work on during the next week until meeting again. Homework is given most sessions to support generalization of learning.

Clinician notes:

- The clinician notes provide detailed information about the outline for each session. The clinician notes are most beneficial if read prior to the session. The clinician notes include each of the following sections:
    - Introduction/assessment:
        - Relationship-building questions and prompts are included to build upon the general framework established in the outline section of the introduction/assessment. Further opportunities to support building rapport are included in this session along with prompts to support gaining more knowledge of the student.

- o Main lesson:
    - ■ Additional ways to support student learning and understanding of new content are discussed as well as explanations of how best to support the growth of understanding. In addition, further explanation is given about why certain activities are completed. This section also provides some further opportunities to tailor learning to the student's age and learning needs.
- o Wrap-up:
    - ■ Explanation is given regarding how to support continued understanding of content covered during the session.

Teacher/guardian summary:

- This teacher/guardian summary is designed to allow for a copy and paste option to easily share learnings from each week with teachers and guardians of the student. Where specific information is needed, there are blanks for the clinician to complete. This section is important in supporting the generalization of content so that learning continues to be reinforced in the classroom and at home. Guardians and teachers are also provided with tools for how to best support students when they are struggling with worry. You'll notice that this section includes a lot of recommendations to share your own experiences as a way to normalize discussing tough situations. Modeling is also used as a way to support reframing thoughts. The intention of self-disclosure and modeling is to support in normalizing the practices being taught.

Chapter 14 Explained

Chapter 14 offers additional support options for the classroom. This chapter provides generalization strategies to help students with worry. Ideally, teachers of students in this group can be provided with some or all of these strategies as a way to continue supporting worry even after completion of the group. However, this section can also be utilized as the group is occurring. Something to consider is that all students can struggle with worry at some point. Therefore, the lessons in this chapter can be beneficial to the whole group because it allows for normalization of the practices and gives students the opportunity to observe modeling and have coping language reinforced with their peers.

Considering the teaching of the skills provided in Chapter 14, for teachers that are less comfortable with supporting social-emotional learning, the clinician can offer to teach the class the lesson. In addition, the clinician can support the teacher with additional coaching around best practice in worry and supporting student coping. In some cases, if students that have been part of a one-on-one or small group session are comfortable, those students may also want to be a part of teaching their class about the knowledge they have gained related to coping skills and what helps them when feeling worried.

Chapter 14 can also be utilized as supplemental materials for use with classrooms or students who have not gone through the nine-week sessions. Materials to utilize can be determined based on what feels most needed by staff or the student(s) themselves. The clinician can guide the teacher in how many practices might be helpful and in what order may best support the classroom.

Chapter 15 Explained

Chapter 15 provides ideas for continued support at home. Additional generalization strategies are given to guardians to use at home with their children if additional support is needed beyond the nine-week sessions. This chapter can also be used for any student(s) and their families if they have indicated worry but are not participating in the nine-week program. The additional practices are laid out to provide specific information on how to utilize varying calming strategies at home with children and as a family. Clinicians can also support families in determining which practices may be most useful with their children and only provide those activities so as to remain focused and not overwhelm guardians with choices.

5 Week 1: Introduction/Get to Know Each Other

Week 1 Outline

Focus

The main goal of this chapter is to build rapport with the student(s) and help them to feel comfortable with you while reviewing what you will do together during your time each week.

Learning Targets

- Students will gain comfort with the clinician and the weekly plan for working together.

Materials Needed

- Pencil and paper.
- Pencil or pen for student.
- Appendix C – Pre/Post Test.
- Appendix D – Weekly Assessment.
- Game/Activity (options include Jenga, Kerplunk, Coloring/Drawing, Playing Basketball, etc.).

Introduction/Assessment

Introduce this session with a greeting and further explanation of how your time together will look. **"Hello, how are you doing today?"** Pause and respond. **"I brought you here today because** (your teacher, parent, I) **recognized that you sometimes struggle with worry, and we thought it might be helpful to work together to see if I can share some strategies with you to help calm some of that worry you may feel each day. We will be working together every week and will discuss emotions, thoughts, and coping strategies. Before we get started, I want to learn more about you and give you the chance to ask me any questions you have."** Pause for introductions and explanations of why you are working together. Work to build rapport with individualized questions and information that can be asked and shared. Then ask, **"Do you ever feel worried?"** If the student(s) says no, provide examples of things that may support the normalization of worry for that student (e.g., needing to speak in front of the class).

It's useful at this point to have examples from teachers or parents from which the student would easily relate). Once worry is identified, ask, **"What types of things make you feel worried?"** Listen and express similarities to others you've worked with close to their age to help normalize the experience of worry.

Further explain to the student(s), **"Worry is something that is not always bad. It can help us to get things done. For example, if you are worried about how you will do on a test, you might be more motivated to study for the test so that you get a good grade. However, worry becomes a problem**

DOI: 10.4324/9781003324782-5

when it takes over a lot of our mind, when it changes our ability to relax and enjoy something, or when we notice ourselves getting worried about things that are unlikely to happen and it gets in the way of our activities and other thoughts." You may ask the student to think of examples of when worry is helpful and when it is harmful.

Next, say, "I would like you to answer a few questions so that I can gather information on what you already know related to worry as well as understand more about your current feelings around worry." Give them Appendix C – Pre-Post Test. Read the questions aloud and support them with any questions. Share with them, "We will take this same test again once we are done working together so that I can understand if your answers to any of the questions change. Our goal of our time together is to support you feeling less worry, and this measure will help us understand if we are meeting that goal." Next, hand them Appendix D – Weekly Assessment and say, "These next three questions will be given to you each time we meet together so that we can see how your answers may change week to week, and again so that we can see if we are meeting the goal of reducing worry." Read the questions aloud and support them with any of their own questions.

Once the student(s) are done with the assessments, state, "Generally, what you say with me will stay with me unless I am concerned about safety. When concerns of safety come up and I am worried about you or someone else being hurt, I need to tell another adult because it's part of my job to ensure that all students are safe. I will be sharing some general information with your teachers and guardians each week so that they can know what you are learning about during our time together, but I won't be sharing specific things that you share with me, especially if you would like to keep it confidential. (For younger students *explain – which means just between us.*) If you ever have any concerns or questions about this, please let me know."

When working in groups, add, "Because we are sharing private information together, it's important that you agree to not share what is discussed by others in our group outside of this room. Does everyone agree to this rule?" Pause and respond with any questions. Also offer, "Are there any other rules or ideas that you can think of that we should agree to as a group?" If they have further ideas, get a piece of paper and write them down under the title Group Rules. This paper should then be displayed at each future meeting.

Main Lesson

Once the assessments are completed, state, "We are going to play a game together today. In this game we are going to take turns talking about a time when we felt a certain way." Games that could be helpful to get to know students are listed below. Questions that may be asked include: do you have any pets? How many siblings do you have? What is your favorite thing about school? What is your least favorite thing about school? What is a favorite memory of yours? Where is the farthest you've traveled? Where is somewhere you hope to go someday?

- Jenga (before pulling out a Jenga piece, the person whose turn it is needs to ask the person to their right a question. Reverse the order after everyone in the group has a chance).
- Kerplunk (similar to Jenga, before pulling out a stick, the person whose turn it is needs to ask the person to their right a question. Reverse the order after everyone in the group has a chance).
- Building together with magna tiles or Legos (talk while you work and build, ask the student questions about themselves and encourage them to ask questions to you).
- Drawing or coloring together (talk while you create, ask the student questions about themselves, and encourage them to ask questions to you).
- Go for a walk outside and talk about life as you walk.
- Shoot hoops together and each time someone makes a basket they share a fact about themselves.

Wrap-up

Plan for when you will meet again and make sure that it works with both of your schedules and is also agreeable by them (make sure that they are not missing their favorite time of the day). Offer the question, **"Is there anything you'd like us to talk more about next time?"** End by sharing, **"I am excited for the chance to get to know you better and look forward to our next meeting."**

Week 1 Clinician Notes

Introduction

Alter the introduction for this discussion based on your knowledge of the student(s) and their perceived comfort level. If there is already a strong relationship, there's less of a need for an introduction, and questions instead can be focused around checking in with the student and learning more about them. However, if this is the first time meeting each other, it is important to share your role and some about yourself. With all students an explanation about the reason for meeting should be stated because otherwise many children may come to conclusions on their own which may be inaccurate. One of the following explanations of the reason for working together could be shared, *"We are working together because* (your teacher/guardians or both – for group – an adult who cares about you) *have concerns that sometimes you worry and it gets in the way of your goals. I've heard you sometimes have feelings of worry. I think that I can help you come up with some ways to work through those feelings. How does that sound to you?"*

After introductions, the student is asked more about their worry. The reason for this happening early on is so that the student can understand and focus on the reason for the meetings each week. If this is the first time meeting the student, be prepared that the student(s) may not feel fully comfortable yet and therefore may be uneasy about sharing their worries. If working with a group, consider calling on a student that may be most likely to feel comfortable sharing. This allows for others in the group to have an idea of what to say, while feeling comforted by the idea of someone else feeling worried and acknowledging this in front of others. If working one on one with a student, an example could be shared related to something they worry about, but is not tied to them as a person. For example, *"For some students I see they worry a lot about getting sick at school. They worry about the germs that others have and if anyone appears unwell or they've heard that someone has been home sick, it takes over their mind and they have a hard time focusing. Has anything like that ever happened to you?"* If the student still says no, it's ok to continue on and encourage them to think over the next week about what makes them feel worried and remind them that we all feel worried sometimes. After sharing about this example of worry, the practitioner should focus on how worry can be helpful. An example might be, if feeling worried about an upcoming test, there may be more motivation to study for the test. Although many kids should resonate with the idea of worry being support-ive in increasing motivation to study for a test, the example given can also be customized to the student(s) and their personality. It's important to help them in clarifying the difference between good and bad worry. *Table 5.1* provides further explanations that could be used and tailored to the student's age and experiences.

Assessment

When giving the student(s) the assessments, ensure that they understand the questions. Read the questions out loud and provide answers to their questions. You may offer to work individually with students if you are in a group and help them by circling their answer. Working individually with each student may help to better gauge understanding and help the student to feel more comfortable opening up if they do not understand the question. If working individually with students on complet-ing the assessment, make sure to have something for the other students to do while they wait such as coloring or fidgets.

Table 5.1 Worry Table

Worry Focus	Helpful Worry	Problematic Worry / Anxiety
Tests	I don't want to fail the test. I am going to study so I get a good grade.	I don't want to fail. I can't do anything else but study. I need to pause eating and reduce my sleep to study. I can't focus on other things except the test.
Safety	I don't want to get hurt in a car accident. I always buckle my seat belt which offers an added protection when I am in the car.	I don't want to get in a car accident, so I avoid riding in certain transportation vehicles.
Arriving on time	I am motivated to get up from my nice warm bed in the morning and get ready so that I'm on time for the bus.	I am so worried about arriving late for the bus that I avoid going all together.
Weather	Being aware of what is happening with the weather helps me to recognize when I should take shelter and how I should dress.	I notice whenever the clouds are turning gray and become unable to focus on anything except the weather because I am scared there will be a storm that will cause harm to me and my loved ones.
Germs	I wash my hands before eating and after using the bathroom to help reduce germs.	I avoid going to certain places where there will be a lot of people and potential germs. I also avoid touching things and wash my hands very frequently as a way to avoid getting sick. When in a place with others, I can only think about the potential germs.

Further explanation of Pre-Post Test assessment (Appendix C) questions:

1 When I start to worry, my mind can't stop thinking about that worry.

   o Explain – think about the last time you felt worried. What was happening inside of your brain? How much were you able to think about anything besides the worry? On this scale of 1–10, circle whatever seems to explain what was happening in your head during that time with 10 being you could not focus on anything else except the worry and 1 being you were able to think about other things easily and the worry didn't bother your thoughts much. Then there is everything in between on this scale, with 5 being that worry somewhat took over your brain but not all the way.

2 I recognize when I feel worried within my body.

   o Explain – do you ever notice your body giving you a clue that you are feeling worried? For example, I feel worried in my stomach. So, whenever I have stomach pain I consider if I might be feeling worried about something. Think about your awareness of your body as it relates to worry. If you are always aware of the clues your body gives you that you may feel worried, circle 10, then consider the rest of the scale with 1 being you are not aware of any of the clues your body gives you when you are feeling worried or anxious and 5 being that you know some of the clues your body gives you but aren't aware of everything that happens in your body when worried.

3 I know how to calm my body when I feel worried.

   o Think about what you do when you feel upset. Are you able to calm yourself quickly or does it take a while? Are you able to try something that works and helps you to lessen your worry? Do you need help from someone else? Or do you often stay feeling anxious for a long time because it's hard for you to feel calm? An answer of a 10 indicates that you can easily and quickly calm yourself down when feeling worried. A 1 means that you are not able to ever do this on your own and don't have strategies that work for you yet. The rest of the scale is somewhere in between and can indicate that you sometimes can help yourself and sometimes not.

4 I know how to challenge my thoughts.

- o Challenging your thoughts means that you are aware of what thoughts you are having and can think about a way to change them so that they are more accurate and less harmful to you. If you are aware of your thoughts and can recognize when you need to change them and how to change them, you would answer a 10 (for example, I may recognize when I tell myself "I am so stupid for missing that answer on the test" and then change the thought to, "Bummer, next time I will get that answer. I did well on the rest of the questions!"). If you do not recognize what thoughts you are having and only notice your feelings (e.g., I feel worried, sad, or frustrated), then your answer would be a 1. You then would indicate anywhere in between if you sometimes were aware of your thoughts and work to change them, and other times not.

5 I utilize stress reduction/calming practices.

- o Stress reduction/calming practices are things that you use on a regular basis. Meaning you do them a few times a week to help your mind stay healthy. Some things people identify as being helpful in reducing stress are reading, swinging, running around the house, playing a game, and petting an animal. Of course, there are others, but if you do something that reduces your stress on a regular basis (a few times a week), give yourself a 10. However, if you never do this, give yourself a 1. If you are still striving to do this more but sometimes use stress reduction practices, mark somewhere in between 1 and 10.

Further explanation of Weekly Assessment (Appendix D) questions:

1 This week I have felt worried…

- o Explain that you want them to think about what has happened over the past week (for younger kids, tie the dates to an event). Remembering all that has happened, think about how much of the time your mind was feeling worried about something. If you noticed this was happening every day throughout most of the day, you would answer with a 10. However, if you do not remember any worry at all, you would answer with a 1. Anything in between might be related to how much of each day you felt you noticed worry, with 5 being half of the time.

2 I recognize different emotions I am feeling during the day.

- o Ask the student(s) if they are aware of different feelings coming and going throughout each day. Do they recognize when their body is starting to feel sad, mad, frustrated, happy, worried, scared, tired? If they are very aware of when they are feeling different kinds of emotions, they should answer with a 10. However, if they are unaware of their emotions unless someone says something to them about their mood, they should answer as a 1. If there are times that they feel aware and recognize "I'm feeling mad right now" and other times are not aware, and someone has to say something or others avoid them "you seem cranky, do you need some space," have them consider the rest of the rating scale.

3 I have been using calming tools when I start feeling worried.

- o Ask the student(s) to think about the different times during the last week they've felt worried and then how they responded to that worry. Do they feel like they have a good plan and can quickly calm themselves? If so, they should mark themselves as a 10. If they struggle to think of ways to calm themselves down and their mind continues to think and focus on worry each time, they should mark themselves with a 1. Anywhere in between should be elsewhere on the rating scale.

When reviewing that certain information will be shared with guardians and teachers, you offer an example of what kind of information will be shared. It's important the student(s) doesn't withhold information because they are worried about what will be shared with others. Explain that in addition to the worry of them being harmed or someone else getting hurt, information will be shared about what the group has learned and the focus of the group so that their guardians and teachers can also help them during the rest of the week. Share that our time together is limited and it's important they practice what was learned even when we are not together. Ask if there is any worry that they have about information being shared with teachers or guardians. It can also be explained that if they ever have this worry come up regarding wanting something they said to be confidential, to share this concern so that a plan can be created that feels good. As the student(s) leaves your room, show happiness about meeting with them next week and offer options of support in case anything comes up in the meantime (e.g., how they can get in touch with you or another mental health professional if they are feeling stressed and unable to handle this worry on their own).

As you discuss group rules with the students that are a part of a group, ensure that they are fully in agreement with whatever is shared in the group stays with the group. It is important that everyone is respectful of this guideline because if they aren't, there will likely be more feelings of worry and less sharing during group time. In addition, look to the students for additional ideas on how the group can feel more comfortable. Students may come up with such thoughts as: don't interrupt when someone else is speaking, show kindness toward others when they are sharing something personal by listening with your eyes and possibly offering a supportive statement like (that must be so hard or I've felt that too), or being open during your time together to share.

Main Lesson

The game played in this session is intended to help in building rapport. During the time together, don't push too much if the child isn't ready. Follow the student(s) lead in terms of what they feel comfortable sharing. Take opportunities to share some about yourself and possibly others that you've worked with that have struggled with worry (while keeping anonymity). If the student(s) aren't into games, check with them on something else they may enjoy doing together. Other suggestions might be to go for a walk, shoot baskets, or play with fidgets together and let them explore your space.

While talking with the student(s) during this session, ask them questions that help in learning more about them as a person and not just their worry. Light humor can be used as it feels appropriate and small details can be shared about yourself. It's important that they see you as a human who also experiences worry so that they can build that relationship but also that they not have too many details shared so that they don't feel a need to be a caretaker and work to be pleasing with their response during each week together. For example, it would be completely appropriate to share about pets, "*I have a cat and her name is Teddy. She makes me giggle when she hops on me to wake me up each morning.*" However, it is not necessary to share a tragic experience surrounding anxiety. This type of sharing could also make the student(s) feel that their worry is not as important or as valid. It is best to not share too much personal information and keep any sharing to a surface level while still gaining rapport.

Wrap-up

Check in with the student to see if there's anything additional they'd like to share before you are done (pause, listen, and respond). Then, as you finish your time together, discuss the plans for when you will meet with the student(s) and make sure that they agree with the time of day and place. It is especially important that this is considered for kids that worry as they may stress about missing certain times in the day. Work to understand what their favorite and least favorite part of the day is and use that information as you also collaborate with their teacher(s) on a time that can work best. Although in the school day, lunch time is often an easy time to meet, consider if you'll have enough time with the number of transitions needed (getting lunch, taking lunch tray back) and the time needed for student(s) to eat and their desire to be social with their friends at this time. If the school offers a scheduled intervention time in the day, that may be a good option if the student(s) isn't already pulled for another group. In addition, it is helpful to consider how meetings will begin. Some students are very worried about how others see them, and they may prefer that they are not seen with you by their peers. Therefore, you may come up with an option together for them to secretly meet (of course the teacher would also need to be aware of this plan). Some plans that may work is to call down to the student's classroom when it is time for them to come and they just come on their own. Or the student may just sign out independently and come to meet. Whatever option is decided upon, make sure that there is a plan for the practitioner or the teacher to remind the student when it is time for the meetings so that the responsibility to remember does not lie with the student.

Teacher and Guardian Summary

Today we worked on getting to know each other by playing a game together. I shared with _____ that we will be working together to support his/her/their worry. Today _____ also took a few surveys so that we can have some information on how our time together may be supporting any changes in emotions and coping. Next week we will begin talking more about emotions including what it's like to feel sad, excited, worried, happy, frustrated, and ashamed.

Homework

It would be helpful if you could check in with your child/student about their thoughts on how today went. Throughout the week, you can introduce a discussion around naming times that you may notice yourself or them feeling sad, excited, worried, frustrated, happy, and disappointed (e.g., ugh, that car just cut me off and I feel frustrated!). If you have a chance, I would love it if you could share these examples that you discuss with your child/student with me as this will help our discussion next week!

6   Emotions

Week 2 Outline

Focus

The main idea of this chapter is to get the student(s) comfortable with explaining and identifying emotions. In addition, there is also a goal to introduce the student(s) to simple breathing strategies.

Learning Targets

- Students will be able to identify and describe different emotions.
- Students will gain awareness in breathing strategies as a technique to relax when feeling worried.

Materials Needed

- Group rules (if applicable).
- Pencil and paper for notes.
- Pencil or pen for student.
- Appendix D – Weekly Assessment.
- For Children: Beach ball with emotions written onto each color (Sad, Excited, Worry, Happy, Frustrated, Shame).
- For Adolescents: Paper and drawing utensils
- Appendix E – Emotions Worksheet.
- Appendix F – (C or A) – deep breathing choices have enough to supply each student with two worksheets.

Introduction/Assessment

"It's so great to see you again, tell me about your week." Pause, listen, and respond. Ask, **"Do you have any questions since we last met and talked about what we'll be doing together each week?"** Pause, listen, and respond. Then, ask the student to complete the weekly assessment (Appendix D).

Main Lesson

For children (beach ball activity): **"Today we are going to throw a beach ball back and forth. You'll notice that I have emotions written on each of the different colors on the beach ball. When I throw the ball to you, pay attention to which color/emotion your right thumb is on. Your job is to then share about a time when you felt this emotion or about a time when you witnessed** (or saw) **someone you know feel this way. We can add fun rules if you'd like or keep track of points. Do you have any ideas to add to this game?"** Pause, listen, and respond. Take a moment to show them the beach ball and ask for their definition of each of the emotions on the beach ball. Play this game for about 10 minutes, taking turns giving examples back and forth.

DOI: 10.4324/9781003324782-6

For adolescents (talking/drawing activity): **"Today we are going to talk about examples of times when you have felt different kinds of emotions."** Give the student(s) Appendix E – Emotions Worksheet. **"I want you to consider each emotion listed on this worksheet and share an example of a time when you felt this way. Consider how your body felt, and what types of thoughts may have been running through your mind. On this sheet, you can write about the experience, or you can draw a picture."** If you have a group, divide the emotions so that they each have one or two. If you are working individually with a student, support them in talking through the examples or allow them to draw an example for each emotion. Once they are finished, have them take turns sharing out their examples to the group.

For both the children and adolescent activities, the following examples and definitions can be used to further explain the emotions:

- **Sad:** to feel down. When you are sad, you feel unhappy, your body may feel low in energy, and you may cry or feel a lack of interest in doing anything.
- **Excited:** to feel intense energy and interest in something. When your body feels excited, it may have a hard time settling down and focusing. Sometimes you may be looking forward to something happening when you feel excited.
- **Worried:** to worry means that your mind is feeling scared about what might happen. Sometimes when you are worried about something, it can be hard for your brain to stop thinking about whatever you are worried about.
- **Happy:** to feel good and glad. Happiness tends to occur when you are feeling calm.
- **Frustrated:** to feel mad about something that may be tough to change or solve. You may feel frustrated when you can't figure out how to solve the math problem.
- **Shame:** to feel pain and like you are less than others. We may feel shame when someone tells an embarrassing story about us to others. We may also experience shame when we feel like others understand something that we do not.

After you are finished, explain, **"It was so nice getting to know you better. Something that is important to remember is that these emotions are ok and normal to feel sometimes. What's important is that if you become stuck in an emotion, you know some strategies to help get you out. Something we can try is a calming activity. Is there anything that you notice that helps you to feel calm?"** Listen and take note of anything that they describe as being especially helpful.

Children: **"Here are some other ideas of strategies that may help you to feel calm."** Share Appendix F-C – children: calming strategies. Review each picture and explain how to utilize it with the child.

4-7-8 Breathing

- **Breathe in for a count of 4.**
- **Hold for a count of 7.**
- **Breathe out for a count of 8.**

Finger Breathing

- **Hold one hand out with fingers open and take the opposite hand's pointer finger.**
- **Trace the open hand by starting on the outside by the thumb.**
- **Take your pointer finger up to the top of the thumb and breathe in, and then breathe out while going down the opposite side of your thumb.**
- **Continue this motion breathing in when going up the next finger and then out when going down until you've traced all the fingers.**

Belly Breathing

- Hold your hand on your stomach and slowly breathe in through your nose, feeling your hand rise as your belly expands.
- Then slowly breathe out and feel your belly shrink back.

Adolescents: *"Here are some other ideas of strategies that may help you to feel calm"* Share Appendix F-A – adolescents: calming breathing strategies. Review each picture and explain how to utilize it with the adolescent.

4-7-8 Breathing

- Breathe in for a count of 4.
- Hold for a count of 7.
- Breathe out for a count of 8.

5-4-3-2-1 Grounding

- Take a deep breath in through your nose and out through your mouth, name 5 things you can see.
- Take a deep breath in through your nose and out through your mouth, name 4 things you can touch.
- Take a deep breath in through your nose and out through your mouth, name 3 things you can hear.
- Take a deep breath in through your nose and out through your mouth, name 2 things you can smell.
- Take a deep breath in through your nose and out through your mouth, name 1 thing you can taste.

Head Stretch

- Grab your right ear with your left hand and gently pull your head toward your left shoulder. Take three deep breaths in and out.
- Grab your left ear with your right hand and gently pull your head toward your right shoulder. Take three deep breaths in and out.
- Take both hands and place them on the back of your head. Gently tilt your chin toward your chest. Take three deep breaths in and out.

Wrap-up

"Over the next week, I would like for you to practice recognizing when your emotions shift and how that feels within your body. Notice what thoughts come up for you. Recognize when your emotions become too big, or your thoughts become challenging. Use a calming strategy and notice how that impacts your thoughts and body sensations. Now, let's end our time together by choosing one of these calm breathing strategies." Send the calming strategies with the student(s) and offer to have one that they can keep at school and one to take home.

Week 2 Clinician Notes

Introduction/Assessment

Make sure to have the group rules sitting out that were agreed upon at the last session if you are working with a group. As you ask the student(s) about how their week has been, check in to see if they've had any worries come up. Listen to their worries and express appreciation for them sharing their thoughts with you. As they complete the assessment, continue to offer to read it aloud for them and walk them through responses as needed. For both the child and adolescent lessons, the objective is to get the student(s) thinking about different types of emotions and be comfortable sharing about situations that make them feel different ways.

Main Lesson

Children's activity: in addition to writing the different emotions on each side of the beach ball, you could also add faces that show the emotions. The games' objective is to get the child thinking and becoming comfortable sharing about times when they may have felt these emotions. After going through the definitions of the emotions as explained in the Session 2 outline, explain the rules to the child and ask if they want to add any fun additions (e.g., if you let the ball bounce, you need to share two examples; you have to throw the ball after spinning in a circle; points can be earned for certain colors and the objective is to get the most points). If you note that the child may struggle with opening up about their own experiences of feeling these ways, offer that they can share about a time that a family member or friend felt this emotion instead. Focus on building trust and comfort throughout the game. Don't push too hard, and if the child gets stuck, help them with examples that you may have heard from their teacher/guardian or your own examples.

Adolescent activity: as the emotion worksheet is shared, consider how the student(s) may feel most comfortable in sharing their examples. Some students prefer to talk, others do better with drawing or writing. Options can be offered to the student such as a choice to talk through three examples, drawing three examples, or writing three examples.

Examples that could be used to further explain the emotions are:

- *I felt sad when my dog died.*
- *I felt excited when I found out we were getting a snow day!*
- *I felt worried when my dog got out of the house.*
- *I felt happy when I got to play outside with my family.*
- *I felt shame when I lied to my parents.*
- *I felt frustrated when I couldn't figure out the recipe.*

When you explain the calming strategies, walk through each of them with the student(s) as they are described by practicing them together. Go-over each strategy together at least twice. For further understanding, you may ask the student(s) which strategy is their favorite and then ask when they might want to try this strategy (in what circumstances might it be helpful). As you identify this plan for trying a strategy, encourage the student to think about how they will recognize the need to try this strategy, whether they will leave their space to try the strategy (e.g., stay sitting or leave the room) or if they will need anyone else to support them in trying this strategy.

Wrap-up

For younger students, it is especially helpful to ensure that their teacher and parents have the copies of the visuals – Appendix F (C and A) – and know which calming strategies are most preferred by their student so that they can encourage the use of this tool. The offer may be made to talk about these different breathing strategies and emotions to the whole class. The lesson could be led by you or the student. If a classroom lesson is able to be given, it would help with generalization of the learning and support the student in seeing others show awareness and acceptance of different kinds of emotions and encourage the use of coping strategies throughout the day.

Teacher and Guardian Summary

For children: today we worked on becoming familiar with different emotions by playing a game. The emotions we discussed were sad, excited, worried, happy, frustrated, and shame. None of these feelings should be talked about negatively, but rather they should be described as a range of emotions that all of us feel. In addition, calm breathing choices were introduced as a tool that can help when emotions feel like they are getting too big and out of control. Strategies explained were 4-7-8 breathing, belly breathing, and finger breathing. I've shared a copy of these strategies with your child with further explanation and visualization.

For adolescents: today we discussed examples of different emotions by sharing about times where situations brought on these different feelings. The emotions discussed were sad, excited, worried, happy, frustrated, and shame. None of these feelings should be talked about negatively, but rather they should be described as a range of emotions that all of us feel. In addition, calm breathing choices were introduced as a tool that can help when emotions feel like they are getting too big and out of control. Strategies explained were 4-7-8 breathing, 5-4-3-2-1 breathing, and head stretching. I've shared a copy of these strategies with your child with further explanation and visualization.

Homework

Throughout the week, help to reinforce reflecting on feelings by checking in and asking your child/ student how they are feeling and talking about your own feelings as well. It would be especially helpful if you could give examples of times when you may be feeling emotions that have the potential to make you feel out of control (e.g., I was so excited about the weekend I had a hard time focusing on work today). Shame is also a word that is not often spoken about much and it would support learning if you had discussions about the meaning of shame and examples of it in everyday life (e.g., what does shame mean to you? How can we become more aware of when we are feeling shame?) Potentially offer a story about them from when they were younger (e.g., when you were little, I remember you locked us out of the house once and I was very upset when you finally let us in. You started to talk badly about yourself as a person and I recognized this was due to shame. We talked a lot that day and I let you know I would always love you but may not always agree with your choices. This helped the shame feeling to get smaller as you recognized that there was nothing wrong with you but rather that it was just a poor choice made and we all have those moments of poor decisions from time to time). In addition, please continue to ask your child/student about the calm breathing choices and encourage the use of these strategies when you notice they are feeling intense emotions.

7 Our Body and Our Thoughts

Week 3 Outline

Focus

The main focus of this section is to integrate emotions with feelings in the body and thoughts that arise. Students gain an awareness of signs that their body gives them when they begin to feel worry and also recognize how to become mindful of their thoughts.

Learning Targets

- Students will be able to identify physical cues related to anxiety.
- Students will be able to explore their thoughts when recognizing they are feeling anxious.
- Students will be able to understand current coping strategies they utilize.

Materials Needed

- Group rules (if applicable).
- Pencil and paper for notes.
- Pencil or pen for student.
- Appendix D – Weekly Assessment.
- Appendix F – C or A – deep breathing choices for children (C) or adolescents (A) (as appropriate based on the age and needs of your student(s). Have enough to supply each student with two worksheets.
- Enough blank pieces of paper for each student along with crayons or colored pencils.
- Appendix G – Worry Sheet (for children).
- Journal (optional).

Introduction/Assessment

"Hello, how have you been doing since our last meeting?" Pause, listen, and respond. Ask the student to complete the weekly assessment (Appendix D). **"I am curious if you noticed any of the emotions occurring in your body that we discussed last week."** Listen and respond. **"Were there any moments where you found it useful to use one of the calming strategies we learned?"** If the student responds yes, ask *"tell me about that time."* If the student responds with no, say, *"Were there times you could have tried using a strategy but just didn't?"* Pause, listen and respond. Support them in their thinking process to reinforce generalization of practice.

Main Lesson

"Today we are going to be talking more about worry within our body. Have you ever noticed your body begins to feel different when you worry?" Pause, listen, and respond. If further explanation is needed, say, *"By this I mean, do you notice that your heart may race, your hands may sweat, your legs may*

DOI: 10.4324/9781003324782-7

shake, your jaw may clench, or you feel some other form of physical response when your brain starts to think about something that makes you feel worried?" Listen to their responses and validate their feelings before continuing. State, **"What we are going to be doing is thinking about a time where you felt worried. If this brings up intense feelings for you, I want to offer that you can leave this space and sit outside the room or choose a calming option within my room."** Have coloring, puzzles, and fidgets available. **"I will get you when we are ready to start again if you leave. If this exercise does bring up intense feelings for you that you'd like to talk through more, please stay after and we will identify some strategies to support you in coping."**

For children: **"I would like for you to think about a time when you felt worried. I have blank pieces of paper here for you to draw what that looked and felt like for you. You can use crayons, colored pencils, or a pencil. As you are drawing, I want you to think about what you remember from the situation and place where you felt worried."** As their drawings begin to come together, say, **"Thinking about that moment where you were worried about something, remember back to how your body felt. Did you notice any certain parts of your body that seemed to be working differently? Just like we talked about a few moments ago, you may have noticed your heart racing, your hands sweating, your legs shaking, your jaw clenching, or something else happening in your body that helped you to know you were feeling worried."**

Hand each student Appendix G – Worry Sheet. **"Thinking about this time where you felt worried, I want you to take a moment to fill out this sheet by circling where in your body you felt the worry. You can circle right on the drawing."** Pause, allow them time to complete this step. **"Now consider what thoughts were in your head when you felt worried and write those thoughts in the thought bubble."** Give the student(s) time to complete this step and support them with prompts of your own thinking if needed – e.g., *"I felt worried when I was running late. My stomach began to hurt and my muscles started to get tight. Thoughts I had were that if I was late I might miss something from class." "Finally, let's write down how you made the worry stop."* You may prompt them to write this or write for them. **"We are all different and therefore may experience worry differently. There is no right or wrong way for how you feel worry. I notice that when I get worried, I start to feel the muscles in my shoulder get tight and that starts to make me have a headache, sometimes I also notice my stomach start to hurt and my jaw clenching."** Ask the students to think, **"Have you ever considered your worries in this way? How did it feel?"** For a group – after the student(s) are done completing the sheet, give them the option to share the worry sheet out loud. If they'd prefer not to talk in the group, they can instead give their sheet to you privately. As they are sharing the worry sheet, prompt students that if they are comfortable to describe the situation in which they felt worry so that the group is provided with some background.

For adolescents: **"I want you to think of a time that you felt worried. Before you tell me about that time, we are going to try something that might feel a little bit scary. However, I want you to remember that I am here and you are safe. Take a deep breath and close your eyes or gaze slightly downward. Think back to this time that you started to feel worried, consider when the worry began and what was around you. What do you see?... Smell?... Feel?... Hear?... Taste?... Once you have the picture of when you began to worry, take a deep breath in and out. Now, think about how your body felt. Where in your body did you feel the worry? Did your stomach feel sick?... Did you notice tension in your shoulders or arms?... Did you feel your face start to get red or your cheeks begin to clench?... What did this worry feel like for you?... Now, take another deep breath."** Breathe in... and out... with them. **"What thoughts begin to come into your mind as you revisit this worry?... What kinds of things did your worry make you start to think about?... Now, take another deep breath. Consider, what happened that made you stop worrying, or forget about the worry?... Take one more deep breath in while counting to four, hold your breath in for a count of seven, and slowly breathe out for a count of eight. Let's do it together, breathe in – one, two, three, four... hold – one, two, three, four, five, six, seven... breathe out – one, two, three, four, five, six, seven, eight. And now, open your eyes."**

"Thinking about what we just practiced, let's share out where you noticed the worry within your body." Ask the student/s or have them take turns and discuss while working with a group. **"Did you recognize a feeling you may not have noticed before?… Or maybe something that's been happening in your body, but you didn't think it was related to your worry?"**

"Our body is interesting because some of the same cues that we have for being physically hurt occur based on our different emotions. These responses can be adaptive because they help our body to prepare for danger and keep us safe. Fight, Flight, Freeze, or Fawn have been identified as ways in which our body reacts against danger. This theory explains that when faced with danger, your body responds in four potential ways: fighting either physically or verbally against the danger (Fight); running away from the danger (Flight); staying still or hiding (Freeze); and responding in a way that is pleasing to someone else to avoid conflict (Fawn)" (Joe, 2021). **"These cues can be helpful when responding to real danger. When we are not in danger, these cues can also be a reminder for us to tune into our thoughts and feelings so that we can work to relax our body."** Offer the opportunity for any questions. **"What did you notice about your body's reaction to stress?… Is this a new awareness for you or something you've been aware of before?"** Discuss any questions/thoughts ideas that come up. After this visualization is finished, offer an opportunity to share, journal, or draw about this experience. Students can share whatever feels most comfortable for them. For journaling or drawing, this can be something that they keep private or share one-on-one with the practitioner. Offer, **"If this experience brought up stress in any way, please stay after with me so that we can talk through options of support."** For students who stay after, offer an opportunity to talk further with you and share coping strategies to support their emotion regulation. Validate this experience and their emotions as they are expressed.

The following are additional prompts to support probing into body clues, thoughts, and coping mechanisms. These suggested questions can be used with both children and adolescents throughout this lesson plan:

1 **Body clues:** "What were the first clues your body gave you that you were beginning to feel nervous?" "Have you felt that way before?" "Did you notice your body feeling this way before or after you figured out that you were feeling worried?" Note that sometimes our body can tell us before our mind.
2 **Thoughts:** "What kind of thoughts popped into your mind?" Consider probing to understand if there were apparent thought distortions happening – all or nothing (I can't believe I missed that shot, I am terrible), overgeneralization (everyone is going to hate me), should thinking (I should be able to do that). Then, challenge that with the student with, *"Was your worry focused on realistic thinking? Or… was it maybe focused on more negative thinking? How likely do you think the worry was to happen? And, if what they were worried about did happen…. How would that feel?"*
3 **What happened to stop the worry:** ask the student, "Tell me more about why the worry stopped." Consider if it stopped because the event they were concerned about didn't happen, because they got distracted, or something else. Ask the student what they learned from this worry and what they might be able to do to try to help calm their body and stop the worry next time.

Wrap-up

Reflect by noting, **"Sometimes when we feel a way other than happy or calm, our body feels shame for feeling that way. Feeling more than just happy and calm can be helpful in making us productive, empathizing with others, and keeping us safe. For example, feeling anxious can push us to prepare to complete something challenging, feeling sadness can help us to gain empathy and perspective to be a more caring person, and anger can give us insight into ourselves and support us in setting healthy boundaries."**

Explain that **"Until our next meeting, I would like you to pay attention to when you are feeling anxious. Notice how your body tells you that you are starting to feel nervous, what thoughts come up, and what**

helps you to stop the worry and feel calm. You can journal these thoughts down (you can offer a fun small journal to share with them) **or you can just keep them in your mind to share with me next time!"**

Week 3 Clinician Notes

Introduction/Assessment

As you ask the student(s) how they are doing, be sure to have the group rules sitting out that were agreed upon during the first session (if working with a group). As you gather information from the student(s), help in supporting the idea of emotions living within the body. This part of the discussion can be connected by explaining that we will be talking more about signals the body gives us that can relate to emotions, especially worry. Recognize that there's often a disconnect between the body and the mind and the focus of this week is to make the student(s) aware of this connection by recognizing different responses that come up for them whether it be thoughts, emotions, or body clues. As it is time for them to complete the assessment, read the questions aloud and touch base on any wonderings that arise.

Main Lesson

Prior to beginning this session, be sure to refer to the guardian and teacher surveys (Appendix B-G and Appendix B-T) to better understand what the student often worries about and what physical complaints are noticed by the guardian and teacher. Having these examples ready will be especially helpful if the child struggles to think of times they've felt worried or where their guardian or teacher notices that they feel the worry within their body. If you recognize that the student simply isn't ready to share feelings of being worried, or that they are struggling to connect with their worry, share a made-up example of someone that shows signs similar to how their guardian and teacher described the worry that the student experienced. After sharing this example, the question can be asked, *"Have you ever felt worried in this way and noticed it in your body?"* If using examples from the Guardian or Teacher Assessment, be cautious with how you share out possible examples and thoughts. For instance, the student may lose trust if they feel that there have been discussions about them that don't include them. Therefore, using an example that you believe they can relate with is helpful. However, saying an exact example given from their teacher or guardian and then stating that you heard this is a worry of theirs may create resistance in sharing more.

Throughout this session, be cautious about how the student is responding and offer opportunities for them to leave the room if they do not feel comfortable. In addition, during times when students are asked to share, always provide the alternative option for them to write or draw instead and for you to instead look at their responses privately. This session may feel vulnerable and it's important to not push the student too much, especially around peers. For students who do not feel comfortable, follow-up with them later on and support them with identifying coping strategies and talking through their stress.

For adolescents: as the student(s) is set up for the visualization activity, make sure to notice and focus on what is most comfortable for them. Some people like to close their eyes, while for others, this can be challenging and lead to more worry and fear. Therefore, open the activity by letting the student know that they should find a comfortable seating position and they can choose to close their eyes or gaze downward at the floor while listening. While reading, pause and read slowly to give the child time to think about this worry in detail and focus on your voice. It is important to try to do this activity in a space that is low in distractions.

While discussing how the body carries emotions, the session shares a further example of "fight, flight, freeze, or fawn" and how these can be adaptive responses when faced with danger. Check in with students if time allows to see if they can think of times when they have recognized one or more of these responses being used by themselves or from someone else. Expand upon how emotions live within the body and if there is a struggle in working through stress (which is part of the coping we will be talking about), the stress may continue to live within the body and show up as physical symptoms.

While completing this activity, if the student(s) describe not feeling any specific body space being impacted this time, ask them about another time they were worried and what it felt like. A specific situation may be prompted to get the student(s) thinking, "*How did you feel on the first day of school? Do you remember where you felt it in your body?*" Personal feelings can then be shared (e.g., "*On the first day of school, I felt nervous and excited because I knew that new people would be around – new students and new co-workers, and others I hadn't seen in a while. I could tell in my body that I was nervous because my stomach began to feel sick and my teeth started to clench. I could tell I was excited because my heart was racing*"). Another option may also be for them to notice where they've seen others show worry as this can help them to feel less vulnerable. Sharing an example about others can also help the student to recognize they are not alone in feeling this way.

As thoughts and their relationship to emotions are discussed, have the student(s) share what kind of thoughts were in their head during this stressful moment. Offer examples such as, "*When I am worried about speaking in front of a group, my mind is thinking – what if you say the wrong thing and everyone laughs at you?*" Examples that relate thoughts to emotions can also be offered, "*If I am thinking about making a mistake, how am I likely to feel?*" (student will likely respond with – worried, scared, nervous). Validate this response by saying yes and sharing with them about how thoughts can really create the types of emotions that we experience. Student learning can be furthered by suggesting that student(s) consider what kind of a thought in their situation may be more adaptive and helpful (e.g., giving a speech in front of others – I will be able to practice in a safe environment where I know everyone). Listen to what answers the student(s) come up with and if needed, support them in prompts that are more positively stated and focused.

After discussing thoughts, move into talking about how calming strategies can be used as a tool to re-set thoughts. Ask questions of them about the types of calming strategies they are most drawn to (e.g., creativity, writing, movement, talking, etc.). Show appreciation for their ideas by opening up about these activities and then share that with the breathing exercises, the reason that these are taught to students is so that they can get better at taking a moment to be still, focus on their awareness of what is happening in the present moment, and to make them aware of the science behind breathing. Explain, "*Breathing deeply helps to ensure that the oxygen we need gets to all the different parts of our body so that we can think, move, and feel calmer. Without deep breathing, when we are anxious, we often breathe very shallow and this can impact our health such as thinking, moving, and general mood.*"

For children: use Appendix G Worry Sheet and ask the child to circle on the person where in their body they noticed the feeling of worry when doing the visualization activity. If the student(s) note that they did not notice any specific body space being impacted this time, ask them about another time they were worried and what it felt like. Having them consider a specific situation may support their thinking, such as, "*How do you feel when a test is handed out?* or "*Do you remember where you felt that emotion within your body?*" After the student shares themselves, provide them with another example (e.g., "*When I am given a test, my whole body tenses up and my heart starts to race. Or, I've heard of other students feeling sick to their stomach whenever a test is given and then it's hard for them to concentrate*"). Another option may also be for them to notice where they've seen others show worry as this can help them to feel less vulnerable, and also promote a sense of awareness that others feel this way and they are not alone. If considering others and how they show worry, utilize real life examples, YouTube, or books. Then ask the student(s) to either circle or color in the parts of the body where they notice their worry.

Regarding thoughts related to emotions, ask the child to draw or write their thoughts within the thought bulbble. Once they're finished, ask them to talk through these thoughts. It's important to see how their thoughts may have contributed to the anxiety. Consider if the thoughts included any possible thought distortions. Help the child to notice how this thought may be more negative and unrealistic in nature and then support them to consider a more realistic possibility. Working through worry in this way will often help children to notice that their fear is unlikely to happen or that it is in fact a thought distortion and not something that is happening.

Finally, as you discuss how the student stopped their worry (or maybe it hasn't stopped yet and you need to talk with them about options on how to stop the worry), ask them to note these feelings of how the worry was stopped, or can be stopped, in the bottom rectangle (Appendix G). Here is where a better understanding of supportive coping tools can be gained. Probe into coping strategies more by asking questions to better understand what they enjoy and how accessible their options are throughout the day. Share the deep breathing choices (Appendix F) and ask them which breathing practice they'd like to try today.

If you need to support thinking for the student in one of these areas of focus (body clues, thoughts, or calming strategies), below provides additional insight.

- **Body clues:** help the student to connect their emotions to their body. Support them in paying attention to the tension that their body feels when they are worried about something. Examples can be further provided such as *"Our muscles tend to tighten and we might tense up our shoulders which then causes tension in our neck which can lead to a headache."* Explain that being aware of how the body holds tension can help in understanding how to work through this tension – for example, if we recognize we tense up our shoulders when stressed, we can be extra aware of our muscle tension and purposefully relax our shoulders as we notice we are beginning to feel worried.
- **Thoughts:** thoughts can be a challenge to connect with feelings, especially for younger children. It is not abnormal to hear a response such as, "I am not thinking of anything." Therefore, the thoughts may need to be further described by helping the student to continue to think of their thoughts in future scenarios when they are feeling worried. Thoughts and their connection to our emotions can be described as, *"Something that can happen when we're worried is to focus on the possibility of something negative happening in the future."* For example, you could add, *"If I wake up and think – ugh, it's raining outside, it's going to be a terrible day. I am likely going to feel sad or annoyed. However, if I wake up and think – it's raining, that means I get to wear my new rain boots. I am likely going to feel some excitement."* Thoughts impact perception of the situation that can support either positive or negative emotions.
- **What happened to stop the worry:** when asking the student(s) about how they moved on from the worry, have them consider what they did that made them feel calm. Most students may talk about a distraction of some sort – such as playing a video game, watching a show, or reading a book. If a distraction gets brought up, validate that this can be a good way to help re-set the mind, especially when emotions are really high. However, when the worry involves working through a problem, such as not knowing whether you should attend your friend's birthday party or the ball game you're playing in, when both are scheduled for the same night, it's important to encourage the student to come back to problem-solving. Strategies to problem solve can be done either independently (e.g., journaling, thinking about what has worked in the past) or with a trusted adult or peer (talking through options with someone else). A question may be asked about whether the student has considered trying something additional as a way to calm their mind like deep breathing, yoga, or going for a walk. These options in combination with their distraction and talking about it in this way can support them in considering additional coping mechanisms for the future.

Wrap-up

To conclude the time together, discuss how it can be hard to feel something other than happy. Explain that although humans are made to experience many different emotions, sometimes shame is felt when other intense feelings arise. Shame means that we feel badly for having done something wrong. It's important that it is noted that any way of feeling is acceptable and expected! Remind the child that we don't want to get rid of these emotions. The goal of our time together is to help them to feel more in control of their emotions and to find ways to recognize when anxious thoughts are coming so that they can use helpful strategies to calm down.

If you have a small journal or notebook, it would be useful to have this on hand to give to the child during the session to allow them to jot down what they notice of their emotions, thoughts, and body throughout the week. It's often hard to reflect when you are only meeting once per week but if the child can make note in a journal about what they notice throughout the week, this can help them to identify what feelings arise and how they are acknowledging them.

Teacher and Guardian Summary

During today's session, we discussed a time where anxiety/worry was felt. We talked through where this feeling is found in our body *(personalize this piece and share it to help parents and teachers best recognize early signs of anxiety)*. We also discussed the types of thoughts that happen when we start to feel worried and how we can challenge these thoughts (e.g., consider the true likelihood of what we're worried about actually happening). As we finished, we talked about things that help to stop our worry *(identify what the student said helped them)*.

Homework

It would be especially helpful if you can check in with your child/student about how today went for them and share about a time when you yourself felt worried. You might explain that situation further by sharing how you felt it in your body (e.g., I could tell I was nervous because my stomach started to hurt), what thoughts came up (e.g., I started thinking that everyone was going to laugh at me), and what you did to help yourself feel calm (e.g., I took a few deep breaths). You can also help by having open conversations when worry comes up with your child/student and helping them reflect on where in their body they feel their worry, what thoughts they are having, and what they can do to feel better.

Work Cited

Joe. (2021, April 7). "The Anxiety Guide Part 1: What Is Anxiety?" – Braver Planet. www.braverplanet.com, www.braverplanet.com/anxiety/the-anxiety-guide-part-1-what-is-anxiety/.

8 Changing Thoughts and Working through Problems

Week 4 Outline

Focus

The main idea of this chapter is a focus on negative thoughts, which often prompt thinking of the worst-case scenario versus what is most likely to happen. In addition, students are taught to think through problem-solving by analyzing multiple possible responses.

Learning Targets

- Students will gain an awareness of analyzing their thoughts as they relate to emotions.
- Students will gain strategies to reframe negative thoughts.
- Students will be able to identify possible solutions to problems and identify the best option for them.

Materials Needed

- Group rules (if applicable).
- Pencil and paper for notes.
- Pencil or pen for student.
- Appendix D – Weekly Assessment.
- Appendix F – C or A – deep breathing choices for children or adolescents (depending on your student's age and needs).
- Appendix H – Thought Reframing Worksheet (need two for each student).

Introduction/Assessment

"Tell me, how has your week gone? Were you able to reflect on how your emotions interacted with your thoughts and body throughout the week?" Pause, listen, and respond. **"Let's complete the weekly assessment now."** (Appendix D.)

Summarize the worry that you heard from the child while checking in with them, or if a worry was not discussed, ask them to consider a time that they felt worried over the last week. Based on this worry, have them complete the Appendix F Worry Sheet (or talk through the prompts from the sheet for older/more advanced children). Once the child is done, ask them to tell you about this experience. Use prompting questions including, **"Where in your body did you feel that you were getting nervous? Did your body feel the worry before you knew in your mind that you were worried? What thoughts did you have? What helped to make you feel calm?"**

Main Lesson

"Today we are going to dig deeper into your thoughts, and work to understand what kind of thoughts may come up for you when you start to feel worried. Oftentimes when people feel worried, they also

DOI: 10.4324/9781003324782-8

start to think more negative thoughts about themselves, and their thoughts may not be realistic. For instance, a worry I have heard discussed is seeing a friend in the hallway and saying hi to that friend and the friend not responding and continuing to walk. Thoughts might arise around that friend being mad and you having done something wrong. However, in reality, what often has happened is that the friend just did not see that person because they had a lot on their mind. Has that ever happened to you?… Maybe you said hi and didn't hear a hello back?…Or you didn't respond to someone else because you didn't hear them?" Pause, listen, and respond. "We are going to discuss how we can evaluate thoughts and reframe them to be more true."

Introduce Appendix H – Thought Reframing Worksheet and have the student(s) share a thought that came up around worry (possibly a thought that arose during the start of the session). If they are not able to think of their own example, they could share one from a friend or get help in coming up with an example from you. Explain that **"We are going to learn two different ways to work through problems today. First, we'll talk about how to work through thoughts that may be focused on the negative, and what we can do when we are worried about the worst thing that can happen. Sometimes, when our mind is worried, it goes right to the worst-case scenario, so it's important to try and re-train our brains and remind our mind to consider evidence against the worst case happening as well as what the best case could be and what is most likely to happen. Sometimes taking a big deep breath can help us to think more clearly."**

You can provide one or more of the following examples:

Situation: I am scared to talk in front of the class.

- What is the worst thing that could happen?
    - Everyone will laugh at me.
- Now, take a big deep breath in and out and notice your body and mind relax…what evidence goes against this happening?
    - I know what I am supposed to say and am ready.
    - The teacher won't allow other kids to laugh at me.
- What is the best thing that may happen?
    - The other students will like what I say.
- What is most likely to happen?
    - Everyone will listen and not laugh while I speak.

Situation: I am scared of riding in a plane.

- What is the worst thing that could happen?
    - The plane will crash.
- Now, take a big deep breath in and out and notice your body and mind relax…what evidence goes against this happening?
    - Planes rarely ever crash.
    - Every time I've ridden in a plane it has been safe.
    - They check planes to ensure they are safe to ride in.
    - They will cancel or delay a flight if the weather isn't right to fly.

- What is the best thing that may happen?
  - I will get to the place I am going and have fun.

- What is most likely to happen?
  - I will get to the place I am going and have fun.

Situation: I am scared I'll fail the test.

- What is the worst thing that could happen?
  - I will have to repeat this grade.

- Now, take a big deep breath in and out and notice your body and mind relax…what evidence goes against this happening?
  - I study hard and have never failed.
  - If I fail one test, my other grades will help me to still pass the class.

- What is the best thing that may happen?
  - I will get an A on the test.

- What is most likely to happen?
  - I will do well and get an A or B on the test because I've studied.

Further explain the worksheet by breaking down each question.

1 **"What is the worst thing that could happen?"** This is a chance for the student to explain what is driving their fear. Work to understand what it is that they are worried about. Discuss with the student how possible this is to happen versus how probable or likely. If the event is possible, it could happen but may be unlikely. Note that in some events, the worst thing could happen, in that case, the conversation needs to change to focus more on supports that would be available should this worst thing happen.
2 **"What evidence goes against this happening?"** Push the student for more examples of information about why this won't happen. Have students take a deep breath as a way to relax their body so that their mind may also think more clearly. Search with them if needed for resilience factors, relationships, and countering evidence to their worry. Explain that *"Usually we worry about the worst case happening, but when we really look at the data, it's very unlikely that this will actually happen."*
3 **"What is the best thing that can happen?"** Have the child fantasize about what good may come of the situation/event/thing they are worried about. Push them to consider what this could look and feel like. Ask, *"If everything goes really well, what would that look like?"*
4 **"What is the most likely thing that will happen?"** Have the child think through what they really think is likely going to happen. Talk with them about how this idea makes them feel and whether this still is something they feel worried about versus the worst-case scenario. Say, *"As you think about what is most likely, how does that make you feel? How do your thoughts about the situation change?"*

"Next, we are going to think through options for how to solve the worry that is coming up for us. There is often more than one way to work through a problem so we are going to consider a few different possibilities and decide which choice might work best by looking at this Thought Changing sheet (Appendix H Page 2)." Share with students the next part of the worksheet where they think through possible options to their problem. Encourage them to think through how they could solve the problem. You might have them say out loud their different ideas for options to what could work, or if they are a more independent thinker, have them complete this on their own and then share it with you. While working together through each option ask, **"What would it look like if you were to choose this option? How would that play out, and what would the outcome likely be in this case?"** And then, **"How anxious does the idea of carrying out this plan make you feel?"**

You can provide one or more of the following examples while referencing Appendix H page 2. Cue the student to take a slow deep breath throughout examining the options as a way to help reconnect with their mind and body and calm their thinking.

Situation: I don't know how to tell the teacher that I'm feeling anxious and need a break.

- Option 1:
  - What is one possible option?
    - I can go up to the teacher and let her know that I am feeling nervous and need a break.
  - Most possible outcome:
    - The teacher will say, ok go take a break.
  - Level of anxiety:
    - 3 – feeling nervous about needing to go up to the teacher to ask, not comfortable because I'm still uncertain what they will say.
  - Can I manage this worry?
    - Yes, I can take deep breaths before talking to the teacher.
- Option 2:
  - What is a second possible option?
    - I can be untruthful, and tell the teacher I need to go see the school nurse.
  - Most possible outcome:
    - The teacher will say, ok go see the nurse.
  - Level of anxiety:
    - 4 – feeling nervous about needing to go up to the teacher to ask, and worried about getting caught lying.
  - Can I manage this worry?
    - No, the worry of not telling the truth will bother me a lot.
- Option 3:
  - What is a third possible option?
    - I can raise my hand and ask the teacher during a calm time in class to let me leave the room to take a break. I can also create a plan for future times so that I don't need to raise my hand but instead can use a hand signal, note, or other agreed upon communication to let my teacher know I need a break because I'm feeling anxious.
  - Most possible outcome:
    - The teacher will say yes, please take a break and will be glad to think about a solution for future requests for breaks with me.

o Level of anxiety:

■ 2 – a little nervous to bring this up to the teacher but feeling better because there are more options and I will feel prepared for future times when I need a break.

o Can I manage this worry?

■ Yes, I can take a deep breath, raise my hand, and then talk to the teacher.

You can then further explain the worksheet by breaking down each question.

1 **"What is a possible option?"** This is a time for the student(s) to talk through the different options that are likely playing out in their mind. It is possible that they have many choices in their head but are getting stuck in organizing these thoughts and thinking through how each of them will play out. Help students to write down each thought that they have and not just jump right to whatever their choice option would be. Note the thoughts as they arise in your discussion and respond without judgment, allowing them to think through each possibility using the information they already have about the situation and the people involved.

2 **"What is the most possible outcome?"** Ask your student(s) to consider their option and then think through what is likely to happen if they choose that option. Questions to consider can include, *"How would others respond? Will this be the outcome you are expecting? What will be the impact on you?"*

3 **"What is your level of anxiety?"** Ask the student(s) to think about implementing this choice and then think about how this would make them feel – considering their body, thoughts, and mind. Ask, *"What would your worry feel like if you made this choice?"* and then have them answer their overall rating of anxiety by indicating this feeling on a 5-point Likert scale with 1 being no or little worry, 3 being some worry, and 5 being high and intense worry.

There is no definitive number of possible solutions to work through with your student. Once they are done with thinking through possibilities, ask them to consider which of these choices is most likely to work out best for them, considering a favorable outcome as well as low anxiety in implementation. Once their choice is made, talk about how this plan will be implemented and offer to support them as needed.

Explain, **"Last week we learned to acknowledge and accept the feelings and thoughts that come up while recognizing the impact of feelings and thoughts on the body. This week, we've talked more about an active role in challenging our thoughts and thinking through options to work through worry. How do you think changing our thoughts may relate to changes in our body or our feelings?"** Pause, listen, and respond. If needed provide this example – *"If I was thinking – 'It's going to be a terrible day, I hate snow!' I likely would feel annoyed, and my body might feel lower in energy. However, if I woke up and thought, Yes, it snowed out! I can't wait to make a snowman later. I likely would feel happy or excited and my body would feel more energized and lighter. Similarly, how does it feel to work through problems by remembering that there are options and there is not a need to be tied to just one possibility? Sometimes, the mind gets stuck and forgets about alternative ways to work through something that is bothersome, and writing down choices, thinking through how choices may play out, and then considering how that choice would feel to implement can help in making the best choice in tough situations."*

Wrap-up

Explain, **"Now you understand how to work through challenging your thoughts and considering the best choice. During the next week, write about one situation that is challenging for you, and work through each of these questions discussed today. I am giving you a second worksheet to do this on your own. Bring this sheet back next week so we can discuss how it went. Notice that your situation may require you to challenge your thoughts, it may require you to consider your options and then** choose the best one, or it may require both." Ask the student to choose a calm breathing activity from Appendix F – Deep Breathing Choices before leaving for the day. Explain, "**Talking about your emotions and thoughts can make your worry increase sometimes. It's important to always take a moment to do something calming like breathing so that we can support our body in working through the stress it may be feeling. Please make a choice for which strategy you'd like to use**" *(reference Appendix F – Deep Breathing Choices).* Do the deep breathing choice with them. Remind them to complete their homework (Appendix H – Thought Reframing Worksheet) before next week's session.

Week 4 Clinician Notes

Introduction/Assessment

As Session 4 begins by checking in with the child, make sure that enough time is allowed to let the conversation go to things that may have come up for the student(s) since the last meeting. Check in on how the student(s) are doing and look for opportunities to incorporate what they share during the session. Incorporating natural discussion will make the time together more meaningful and more easily generalized into their everyday life. Also, note that the questions during the session are options of what can be asked to the student, and not all need to be asked. Be careful to pause and follow the student's lead for discussion points. Continue to read through the weekly assessment with the student(s) and support with any questions that come up.

Main Lesson

Prior to this session, it would be helpful to have the guardian and teacher questionnaires (Appendix B-G and Appendix B-T) available to reference for any questions that arise or if the student struggles to think of challenges that come up for them. Reading the questionnaires ahead of time will also help in an understanding of what types of scenarios might be most relevant to the student(s) to use as examples. For instance, if a student(s) guardian largely is identifying that their child most often expresses worry about social situations, then the example in the outline about a person feeling worried about others laughing at them might be most appropriate. If the student's teacher explains that the child is very worried about classroom performance and is always wanting their work to be perfect, the example given in the outline around failing a test would be most relatable. For students whose parents or teacher have expressed specific fears (e.g., storms, fire, heights, etc.), the plane example may be most easily generalized for that student.

Note that throughout this session you are working on teaching the child two new skill sets. One is the skill to recognize negative thinking and challenge that thinking to be more realistic. Negative thinking is challenged by considering whether that case is really likely to happen, what data is available against this negative worry, what is the best-case scenario, and then what is most likely to happen. The second skill being taught is to think through options to solve a problem by considering what choices are available, what it might look like to follow through with each choice, and how anxious each choice may make the student feel. For the session, each of these skill sets will be worked through so that the student is aware of these options when they need them.

When working through the skills, one skill set may be more useful than another. To determine which skill set to use, prompt the student to consider the situation. Is this a case where they are focused on the worst-case scenario? Or is this a case where they need possible options to think through a solution. Be cautious in this session to be aware of worries that come up that are focused on the worst case, but the worst case may be likely to happen. For example, a student who is very worried about their grandpa dying because they are sick. You don't want to provide the student with unrealistic hope that their worries of grandpa dying are inaccurate. However, in this type of a situation, you may instead say, "*This is a tough worry and I understand why it's on your mind. I don't feel like you're being overly negative in your thinking, but I wonder if we can think about possible solutions or ways that you can handle this worry so that it feels more manageable.*" You then can have the situation be: what can I do when I start to think about my grandpa, and work through possible options for this scenario.

Skill Set 1 – Worst Case, Best Case, Most Likely

While working through worries with a student, time may need to be spent supporting the student(s) in talking through their worries to better identify what they are most worried about happening – what is their "worst-case scenario." For example, if a student says I am most worried about storms happening and then say their worst-case scenario is that it will be loud, and the storm will come – ask more. Probe with: "*What are you most worried about happening if a storm comes? What would be the worst thing that may happen if a storm did come?*" This can help ensure that the worst-case scenario is truly understood and not just the surface of their worry. Asking questions in this way will also help the student(s) to better understand what is feeding their worry. They then can pay more attention to their thoughts and what is feeding the feeling of worry which can lead to a response such as, *I'm really worried about the storms coming because I don't want our house to blow away and for me to lose all of the items that I love. I saw this happen on the news before to other families.*

Talking about a fear of what is the worst-case scenario with a student can bring up a lot of stress and anxiety. Offer opportunities for deep breathing to occur if you notice the student is becoming anxious and also as a way to teach them this as a tool to slow their mind and reconnect with their body. While doing this, you can breathe in deeply with them, hold the breath, and then breathe out slowly. Ask them to recognize how breathing in that way changes feelings in their body and mind.

While talking about the evidence that the student has for this worst-case scenario happening, language can include questions surrounding why this worry is unlikely to happen. Instead of evidence, the terms "data" and "reasons why" can be used for younger students. It's important to support the student in this process and ask questions like, "*Has this ever happened before? Has anyone you know had this happen? What have you done already that makes you think your worst case is unlikely to happen?*" These questions help the student to think about what they already know and support them in feeling more confident in their understanding.

As the child considers what is the best-case scenario, support them by thinking within the worry. Use supportive words such as, "*If everything goes better than expected, what would that look like?*" Work to keep them focused on your discussion and ensure that the best-case scenario is related to the topic.

While talking through what is most likely to happen, have the child first review all of what has been discussed. Give a brief summary of each step prior including what they shared was their worst-case scenario, the evidence against this happening, and what would be the best-case scenario. Have them then consider, "*Thinking about all that we've discussed, consider what you think is most likely to happen.*"

While working through personal worries, consider if a student may have a high likelihood of something tough happening for them. For example, a student may express a fear of becoming sick. You could talk through what being sick has looked like for them before by asking about how long they were sick and if they felt all better once they weren't sick anymore. Then, rather than looking at data that shows this is unlikely, have them consider what resiliency factors they have, including people that could support them if their worry were to happen. This section truly is geared toward meeting the student and their worry needs where they are at and then catering a thought reframing plan accordingly.

Skill Set 2 – Possible Options

When supporting the student in possible options to the problem, make sure you initially have the problem clearly identified. For example, if a student says I hate talking to my teacher. Delve into this more with questions such as, "*What is it that you don't like about talking to your teacher? Do you always not like talking to your teacher or just sometimes? – Tell me more. What are you worried about happening when you talk to your teacher? Is it just your classroom teacher or is it all teachers that make you feel worried to speak?"* These questions can help to more specifically identify the problem and concern for the child. Your problem could go from "I hate talking to my teacher" to "I feel scared to ask my teacher for a break when I am feeling anxious because I am scared she will say no."

After specifically identifying the situation, you can then ask the student for potential choices in how they can work through this problem. Be cautious to let the student come up with most of this independently. You may prompt them to bring their awareness to their body as they consider different options, and notice whether the option feels good (body calm) or scary (body tense). Remind them that they know the teacher (or whomever is involved in the situation) best. Based on the knowledge that they already have, they are able to make an informed decision about how their teacher will respond to different solutions. Help to also remind them to consider possible options that may not have been their first idea, just so that they can be compared and thought out similar to other potential choices.

Next, the student is prompted to consider how each possible option to the problem may play out. Sometimes, when feeling anxious, it can be hard to consider multiple perspectives, so the student may be reminded to consider, *"How would other people involved feel about this as a choice? How might this choice impact you and others in the long term?"* To help, you may support the student in a visualization practice where you play out each possible option and have them consider what the response may look like based on these choices. In addition, you can help the student to ground their mind by taking some deep breaths in and out together.

Finally, because anxiety can be a large driving factor in decision-making, have the student think about how each choice would feel for them. Reference them to think about whether they would feel nervous or worried about something involved within the actual choice and then to make their rating based on that feeling. Their level of worry may come from the idea of talking face to face to a person of authority, from speaking up in front of class, from the worry of being told no, or many other things that may weigh heavily on their mind. Considering level of worry helps to tie emotions into the choice and not just what the best outcome would look like.

Once each possible outcome is written down and talked through thoroughly, have the student look at their options and choose what they think is the best solution to their problem. Remind them that there is not a wrong solution, it is just whatever works best for them. Encourage them to consider their thoughts and feelings as well as others' thoughts and feelings, and to choose the choice that they feel will provide the best outcome.

Wrap-up

Offer to support with any questions that may come up as well as thoughts students may have about this activity. Ensure the student understands that you'd like them to try this on their own with one activity over the next week before your next time together. Ask them about their thoughts on where a good place to keep the sheet might be. This prompt is intended so that they don't forget about the task. Also prompt them about considering a good time to reflect on their day and fill out the sheet. Doing this will ensure that the sheet is more likely to be completed. Remind the student that it may feel tricky to think about whether they should choose the Worst Case, Best Case, or Most Likely table, or if they should choose the Possible Options table. Remind them that different problems require different solutions and that if they feel like they are getting stuck on the negative that isn't likely to happen, the Worst Case, Best Case, or Most Likely part of the sheet may be best, but if they are instead uncertain as to how to work through strong feelings or a problem, the Possible Options portion may work best for them. Let them know they also are welcome to do both with one situation or two separate situations with each sheet so that they can get practice!

As the student chooses their deep breathing activity, do their choice with them and remind them that these can be options for them to use when they start noticing themselves getting worried about something and thinking about what the worst-case scenario may be. Further explain to them that calming their brain may help them to then be able to better think through the situation and consider what is most likely to happen. If the child has a journal, its use can be encouraged as a way to record more thoughts and recognize thinking patterns. Practice in this thinking will help to support more likely and more positive thinking.

Teacher and Guardian Summary

Today we discussed how to change worry thoughts that may not be helpful. We first practiced challenging these thoughts by considering: (1) What is the worst thing that can happen? (2) What evidence do you have that the worst-case scenario isn't likely to happen? (3) What is the best thing that can happen? (4) What is most likely to happen? As your student has worries, it would be helpful to guide them with these questions to help to challenge their thinking more and consider alternative thoughts that may be more accurate and helpful. You can also help by modeling this on your own. For example, explaining, "*Today, my friend said she was going to call me and never did. I started to think that she must be mad at me about something and started getting frustrated with myself for not being a better friend. I then changed this thinking to remember that my friend has a lot going on right now and she likely got busy with other things that had nothing to do with being mad at me.*"

In addition to challenging thoughts, we also talked through situations in which strong feelings or worries may come up and we just aren't sure how to problem solve. We identified possible choices that could be taken and then considered what the outcome might look like for each choice as well as how that may make us feel relating to our level of worry. You can work with your child on building this skill by working through a problem together or modeling your thinking (e.g., "*Hmmm, it looks like we have a problem, I was planning on going home right after school to get supper ready, but you were thinking we'd go to the library because we talked about that idea last week. We could – go home right away and have supper which might make you feel a little more anxious because you really want to have a book; we could – go to the library and then go home which may make me feel a little anxious because we'll be eating supper later than I expected; or we could go to the library and pick up something to eat so that we still get books and also get to eat at the expected time which will make both of us feel less anxious. Why don't we go with our third idea and pick up supper after we go to the library?*"). Although our mind often does these things independently, it's good to model all of the thinking components and pieces to consider when planning so that your child can feel more confident in doing this independently.

We continued by going over the deep breathing choices I shared previously. These deep breathing strategies can also be used to help in slowing down and recognizing the thoughts that are coming into their mind as well as the potential choices and their impact on thoughts and feelings.

Homework

Your child/student has been tasked with thinking through a situation that they are worried about and choosing to use one of the tools we learned (or both if they wish). They will do this by identifying what is the worst-case scenario, evidence against that happening, the best-case scenario, and then what is most likely OR identifying possible options to the problem, potential outcomes with each option, and then how each option might make them feel regarding level of anxiety. It would be helpful if you were able to ask them about this sheet and offer to talk through the situation with them.

9 In and Out of Control/Coping Strategies

Week 5 Outline

Focus

The main goal of this chapter is supporting students to feel confident in thinking through problems and identifying what is within their control – referred to as a Play-Doh problems (due to its moldability), and what is outside of their control – referred to as a rock problems (due to its hard unchangeable structure). Students are then introduced to stress reduction practices.

Learning Targets

- Students will be able to understand their role in a problem and what they have the power to change, and then in contrast, understand what is outside of their control.
- Students will be able to identify at least three stress reduction practices that they can utilize when feeling anxious.

Materials Needed

- Group rules (if applicable).
- Pencil and paper for your notes.
- Pencil or pen for student.
- Appendix D – Weekly Assessment.
- Appendix F – (C or A) – Deep Breathing Choices have enough to supply each student with two worksheets.
- Appendix I – Control and Stress.
- Appendix J – Coping Strategies.
- Appendix M – Calming Practice.
- Rock (optional).
- Play-Doh (optional).

Introduction/Assessment

"How are you today?" Pause, listen, and respond. "Did you have moments of stress where you were able to practice considering worst, best, and most likely scenario?" Pause, listen, and respond. "What about times where you instead considered possible options and chose what you felt would be the best choice after thinking through each option?" Pause, listen, and respond. Ask the student to complete the weekly assessment (Appendix D).

Main Lesson

Explain, "Today we are going to be considering how with each worry that comes up, there is a piece that is within our control, and a piece that is outside of our control. For instance, if you feel worried

DOI: 10.4324/9781003324782-9

about a test, it is within your control to decide how much to study, but it is outside of your control as to which questions the teacher puts on the test. Considering problems in this way can help us to think about how much authority we have over our situation. Although we do not have control over other's actions, we do have control over our own actions and our own actions may also influence others as well. For my mind, it helps to consider these problems in the terms of Play-Doh – the pieces that I can easily mold and change because they are within my control (while saying this hold and squish playdough) and rock problems – the pieces of worry that are outside of my control and cannot be altered by me" (while saying this, hold rock).

"Let's think about the following situations and identify what pieces are moldable like Play-Doh and what parts are outside of your control and not able to be changed, like a rock." For a group of students, write out each situation on a piece of paper and have each student pick one situation and share their thoughts on the moldable/Play-Doh option and the outside of control/rock piece. If working one-on-one with a student, have them talk through four of the problems out loud (choose whichever situations feel most applicable to them). The answers below are possible choices, but the student(s) may come up with alternative options as well.

- Situation: "*A classmate doesn't invite you to their party.*"
  - Possible answer:
    - Moldable/Play-Doh – the response to their friend and others invited, e.g., still being kind to this classmate and those invited to the party. Choosing something to feel calm.
    - Outside of control/rock – who is invited to the party.

- Situation: "*You are in a fight with a friend.*"
  - Possible answer:
    - Moldable/Play-Doh – a discussion with a friend to try to solve the problem. Choosing something to feel calm.
    - Outside of control/rock – the friend's response to them and the discussion.

- Situation: "*You got a bad grade on a test.*"
  - Possible answer:
    - Moldable/Play-Doh – choices for future tests, or how to bring up the course grade (e.g., asking for a re-take, studying hard for the next test, or doing well on homework). Choosing something to help you feel calm.
    - Outside of control/rock – the test grade and how the teacher will respond to requests to try and improve the grade.

- Situation: "*Your parents are fighting a lot.*"
  - Possible answer:
    - Moldable/Play-Doh – working to not be able to hear the fighting (e.g., going to another space or using headphones). Choosing something to feel calm.
    - Outside of control/rock – parents fighting and what they are fighting about.

- Situation: "*Whether it will storm.*"
  - Possible answer:
    - Moldable/Play-Doh – alternative plans if it does storm. Going to a space where the storm can't be heard. Choosing something to feel calm.
    - Outside of control/rock – if it does storm/the weather.

- Situation: *"Classmates laugh at you."*
  - o Possible answer:
    - Moldable/Play-Doh – the response after classmates laugh, e.g., ignoring classmates, saying something back, and telling a teacher.
    - Outside of control/rock – how classmates respond.

"While considering the control we have over a situation, let's also build upon the body's capacity to remain calm through regular stress reduction practices. Every person has something different that seems to help them with feeling calm. What have you tried already that helps you to feel calm when you notice your body feeling stressed?" Pause, listen, and note what they've stated.

Based on what the student says, probe further about what might be most interesting for them to use as a calming strategy. Share with them the Coping Strategies handout (Appendix J). "I'm going to have you complete the Coping Strategies hand out (Appendix J)" and have them take a moment to circle which of these strategies they would be open to trying. You can offer that they can read them independently or you can read the options aloud while they circle. To describe each section further, you can add:

> **"Does your body enjoy moving to calm down? – yoga, walking, weightlifting, running, and dancing are all some options to support body movement."**
>
> **"Are you someone who enjoys being creative? – using art might be beneficial to working through tough feelings along with other modes like baking, photography, or organizing."**
>
> **"Do you feel like your mind has a hard time settling down and it needs to practice being more still? – if so, guided mindfulness or deep breathing can be helpful."**
>
> **"Do you sometimes get stuck with negative thinking and need to have reminders to focus on what you are thankful for? – considering moments of thankfulness, like listening to a guided meditation where someone walks you through a gratitude exercise, can be helpful. Writing or saying three things you are thankful for each day can also work to change your mind to be positive."**
>
> **"Do you do best when you are able to be close to someone? – you may benefit from talking to another person, being near a pet, connecting with another while working to be calm in some way."**

Remind the student, **"There is no one way to reduce stress, the important thing is that we figure out what seems to work best for us and then incorporate this practice into a regular routine."** Don't push them to do something they aren't comfortable trying but offer an opportunity for them to consider a few different strategies that they haven't yet done. Walk through two to three of these strategies with them. They may choose, or you can support them in offering choices based on what you've learned about them and from the parent and teacher questionnaires.

Wrap-up

"Over the next week, I want you to complete this worksheet – Control and Stress Worksheet (Appendix I). **As a problem comes up that causes you stress, write it down and determine which parts are within your control/Play-Doh and which parts are outside of your control/rock as you think through the problem. I would also like you to complete this second worksheet (Appendix M) by documenting your experience trying at least three different choices from what you selected from the Coping Strategies handout** (Appendix J) **throughout the week."** Prompt the student(s) to choose a Calm Breathing Activity from Appendix F (C or A) before leaving for the day.

Week 5 Clinician Notes

Introduction/Assessment

When checking in with the student, consider their examples of the worst, best, and most likely scenario from the prior week. Talk further about their examples and question them by asking them to dig further into their thinking. Help them to consider the accuracy of their statements. If the statements feel inaccurate, say, "*Why might you think that way? What experience do you have that makes you feel that this may be the worst/best/most likely scenario?*" If the student struggles to come up with examples, be prepared to consider examples that would pertain to them. It would be especially helpful if you were able to have additional input from guardians or teachers.

If an example does not exist, use a general example such as, "*What if I am worried about how I will do on a test?*" Then ask that they help you think through what the best, worst, and most likely scenario could be for this situation. If they struggle still with this line of thinking, explain what may be expected at their school. For example, the best-case scenario might be, "*you do well because you've studied hard.*" The worst-case example may be, "*you fail the test, but your teacher allows you to retake it later.*" The most likely scenario then may be, "*they are likely to do well on the test because they are worried about their performance and have studied.*"

Main Lesson

When explaining problems that are within our control (Play-Doh) and problems that are outside of our control (rock), use a visual with your hands. For Play-Doh, show your hands moving like you have Play-Doh, or get out some Play-Doh and ask them if they can form the Play-Doh. This will help students to better grasp the idea of within their control. For outside of our control – rock problems – have a rock with you and ask them if they can break this rock. Ask them to try whatever they'd like but note that they are not able to break that rock with the tools available to them. Therefore, the rock represents those problems that are outside of our control and unable to be changed by us. You could show the rock sitting on a shelf – representing that you are aware the problem is there and acknowledge the problem but know you can't do anything to change the rock.

Further explain that, "*Problems are often complicated or dynamic – meaning that a problem may have lots of different parts and might not simply just be all outside of our control or all within our control. As we remember this, we can recognize what parts of the problem we do have control over and can mold like Play-Doh, and also be aware of those things that are outside of our control, and we can recognize and be aware that they bother us but also know there's nothing we can do if it's something that is outside of our control.*" The following examples can help in further describing each of these ideas. The next steps can be used if the student(s) are ready to further evaluate the problems discussed in this session.

- *A classmate doesn't invite you to their party* – for this example, it is largely described as a rock problem. However, you can further expand upon how they choose to act toward this person and others that are invited to the party. They have the choice to be kind to them even though they are not invited. They also can make the choice to leave the area if the party is being discussed and they don't want to hear about it and feel left out.
- *You are in a fight with a friend* – this problem is largely a Play-Doh problem because you can determine how to move forward with this friend by talking through the situation calmly. You might even ask the student for examples of how they would try to address this friend if they knew they were mad at them. It is important to explain that although they do have control in their response to this situation, they are not able to control how their friend will respond.
- *You got a bad grade on a test* – this problem is largely a Play-Doh problem. It was your performance that led to the bad grade, so you can assess what could be done differently next time and how your grade can be brought up in that class. However, you do not have control over the types of questions that will be asked and how the teacher might respond if you were to ask for an opportunity to retake the test.
- *Your parents are fighting a lot* – with this situation, it is largely a rock problem because you have no way to prevent your parents from fighting, even if their fighting includes pieces about you – you are not able to control what they fight about. However, if you don't like your parents fighting, you can have a plan to leave the space when they are fighting or listen to music or a show, so you don't hear them.

While moving into rating of coping strategies (Appendix M – Calming Practice), know that this is just a general introduction for the student as more detailed explanation and practices will occur in two weeks. This sheet is meant to better understand the student's openness to different forms of coping strategies. In this section, explain any strategies further that the student may not be aware of their meaning. In addition, you may add other alternative options the student(s) mentions are helpful to them but are not listed.

As stress reduction utilization practices are considered, listen to the ideas that are shared by the student. Consider what stress reduction method they seem most drawn toward – movement, artistic/creative, breath work, gratitude, connection. Keeping their preference in mind may help in introducing them to other opportunities to practice stress reduction that they haven't yet tried but are open to trying. The ideas given throughout this session are also just some ideas, of course there are many ways that people may work on stress reduction.

To support buy-in of stress reduction practices, explain to the student(s) that when we experience intense emotions, these emotions can live inside of our body (Nagoski & Nagoski, 2020). Our body then needs some sort of physical release in order to let go of the stress that we just experienced. When we can't have a physical release of some sort, it can lead to us experiencing pain within our body.

While talking about options for the student(s), some may really struggle with the idea of being still with their thoughts. This can be an indicator of trauma or alternative sensory needs. Therefore, if the student(s) is very resistant to some forms of coping, don't push it. In addition, always offer the opportunity for students to leave their eyes open during any type of meditation or yoga practices so that work occurs within their bounds of what feels safe and supportive.

Wrap-up

When sharing the homework plan, ensure that the student(s) understand what is expected and have an opportunity to answer any questions. Note that they will take home both the Appendix I – Control and Stress Worksheet and Appendix M – Calming Practice. For the Calm Strategy Rating, you may offer that they can do three days or more of documentation and offer a second worksheet if they'd like more than three days. Work with the student(s) to determine a time for when they will complete the worksheets. Be specific with the Calm Strategy planning, as this is more likely to ensure practice occurs. Ask them questions like: *"Would it work best if you did this before or after school? … At home or somewhere else? … How long will you take to try a calming practice? … What will you try first?…"* Once finished with this discussion, encourage them to write out this plan on their sheet before leaving. Make a copy of Appendix J – Coping Strategies so that they can reference this sheet when documenting their Calm Strategies and so that you can keep one for your records.

Teacher and Guardian Summary

This week, our discussion revolved around considering what is within our control and what is outside of our control when thinking about a problem. We further identified the components of problems and indicated that when part of the problem is within someone else's control, it is the "rock" of the problem and the pieces that are changeable and something that we can say or do is the "Play-Doh" of the problem. Examples that we discussed include: _____

_____

(Identify some examples that the student(s) especially took interest in talking through.) In addition, we began to identify coping strategies that your student may be interested in trying.

Homework

You can continue to support this learning by checking in with your student when there's a problem and asking them what parts are out of their control (rock) and what parts are within their control (Play-Doh). They have been asked to document this occurrence during the next week. In addition, we identified different ways that may support them when working to reduce stress. I've sent their sheet home with them to share the options they are open to trying and am also asking that they document a few days of trying out different coping strategies and identifying any changes with their feelings after trying out an option. You might try to encourage them to try some of the different calming exercises or ask about how different kinds of practices are working for them. It would also be helpful for you to share with your child what type of practice you utilize to support your own stress reduction.

Works Cited

Nagoski, Emily, and Nagoski, Amelia. *Burnout: The Secret to Unlocking the Stress Cycle.* New York: Ballantine Books, 2020.

10 People That Help Our Thoughts

Week 6 Outline

Focus

In this chapter, students work to analyze their relationships by documenting people that are close to them. They are then challenged with the idea of thinking about how this person influences them – negatively, positively, or both negatively and positively. While considering what is important to them as a person and the people they surround themselves with, students identify a goal for themselves to make a change to better support positive thinking.

Learning Targets

- Students will be able to identify how people in their lives impact them in a mostly positive, mostly negative, or both positive and negative way.
- Students will be able to identify life or relationship changes that they need to make in order to support a more positive well-being for themselves.

Materials Needed

- Group rules (if applicable).
- Pencil and paper for your notes.
- Pencil or pen for student.
- Appendix D – Weekly Assessment.
- Appendix F – (C or A) – Deep Breathing Choices have enough to supply each student with two worksheets.
- Appendix K – Positive/Negative Influences and Relationships
- Appendix M – Calming Practice

Introduction/Assessment

"Hello, how has your week been?" Pause, listen, and respond. "Let's complete the Weekly Assessment Sheet – Appendix D" Once finished, **"Let's talk through your homework."** If the student didn't complete the sheets, take time to work on them together. Ask, **"How did it feel to consider problems by breaking them down into what is within and what is outside of your control?"** Pause, listen, and respond. **"When you began to feel nervous about a situation, how did your body feel? Did you notice those feelings changing within your body as you thought about what was in your control and what was outside of your control?"** If the student struggles to respond to this question, offer an example, *"I notice that when I feel nervous, my shoulder muscles feel tight and my stomach hurts. But when I recognize that I'm able to change how I handle the problem, like by talking through a fight with my friend, and also recognize that I am not able to change how they respond to me, helps me to feel more in control and my stomach hurts less. This isn't always able to work though, and sometimes I need to use a stress reliever practice like going for a walk or taking deep breaths."*

DOI: 10.4324/9781003324782-10

Then, **"Tell me about what coping strategies you tried."** Pause, listen, and respond. **"What did you notice about your emotions? Did they change from before you tried the strategy, to after trying the strategy? Did you learn anything about the type of coping strategies you find most helpful?"** Pause, listen, and respond.

Main Lesson

"During the last few weeks, our time together has focused a lot on what is happening within our body and mind. Can you remember some of the things we've talked about related to worry, our body, and our mind?" Pause, listen, and respond. If they miss anything or need support, add any of the following:

- *"We've discussed how paying attention to our body can indicate feelings of worry."*
- *"We've talked about how our thoughts can impact how we feel."*
- *"We've talked about what is within and outside of our control."*

"Today let's consider how others might influence your thoughts and actions. Do you know what influence means?" Pause, listen, and respond. If further explanation is required, offer, *"influence means how someone impacts or affects your thoughts, feelings, and actions."*

Reference to Appendix K

1st column on left – **"Think about yourself and what is important to you as a person right now. I would like you to especially think about the things that others may not be able to see but would notice when they are around you. What are some things that you might say describe what's most important to you at this point in your life? Some examples might be: honesty, help, kindness, caring. There are many other words that can be used. What words are important in describing you?"** If the student struggles, help them by sharing attributes of them that you have noticed, or others have shared with you about that student. **"I want to also take a moment to mention that these words that are important to you may change as you get older and go through different experiences, and that is ok!"**

Middle column – **"I would now like for you to consider people that you enjoy being around. Think about what they do and how they act that makes you like being around them. We are going to write those ideas in this column"** (point to middle column). **"What characteristics of others help me to feel good?"** Watch and offer ideas/feedback as they think. Write the ideas down for the student or prompt them to write themselves. After at least three examples have been written down, move to the next column.

3rd column on right – **"Great, those are characteristics that would help most people to feel good. Next, we are going to think about what characteristics make you feel bad. These are things that someone else may say or do that are not helpful to you and may negatively impact your feelings. It may make you feel more nervous, sadder, or in some way go against the things that are important to you."** Support the student in coming up with these ideas and talking through why they wrote these down. Wait until three examples have been written down and then move on.

Bottom circles – **"On the bottom of this sheet, there are three circles. The middle circle represents you and all that is important to you as a person and the characteristics that make you, you! This middle circle is people who may influence you. Remember, we talked about how influence means – how someone impacts or affects your thoughts, feelings, and actions. These are people such as your family and best friends who are close to you and you are around frequently. They may influence you mostly positively, negatively, or both positively and negatively. The largest outside circle is people who you have contact with but not someone whom you would share a secret. These might be classmates, someone on your team, or a cousin. Outside of the circle is noted as 'everyone else.'**

These are people who you may run into throughout the day but don't talk with much. These people may include your doctor, a grocery store clerk, or school secretary."

Positive influence – **"As you look at the names of the people you've written down, refer to the top of the page and consider which people on this list are those who help you to feel positive in some way and put a + sign next to their name. For example, if my best friend is always willing to help me when I am feeling sad, I would put a + next to their name."** Help them to talk through this more if needed. Then, give them time to work through which names are + influences in their lives.

Negative influence – **"Next, I want you to look at the top of the page and remember that we wrote when people do ...... (list off what is written), you feel that they are not helpful and may make you feel bad. Look at the names you have listed and decide which people influence you negatively and place a – next to their name. As you are doing this, consider how some people may at times influence you positively and at other times influence you negatively. It's ok to put a – symbol next to someone who has a + already."** Help the student through this activity if it feels they are getting stuck, bring up their negative influencers, and ask if they ever notice anyone on the paper doing these things? You can offer, *"An example of a negative influence might be someone who is always saying hurtful things that make you feel down on yourself."*

Positive and negative influences – once the student has identified all positive and negative influences, ask them to next look at those people that have both a + and next to them. **"Next, I would like for you to look at all of the names you have listed with both a + and – next to the name. Without thinking too long about it, circle whichever symbol you believe is what the person shows most often. As you are doing this, consider if your body gives you any clues as to which symbol is most appropriate for which person."** Talk through this with the student by identifying what you are noticing with what they circle and asking questions about how they determined which symbol should be selected.

Making changes to the circles – once the worksheet is complete, ask the student, **"What do you notice from how you identified the influence of people within your close circle?"** Pause, listen, and respond. Ask them if there might be any changes they could make to their circles. Potential change options may include:

- Moving someone out from the outer circle into the inner circle by building a relationship with them.
- Moving someone out of the inner circle to the outer circle by spending less time with them.
- Working to find more positive influences.
- Leaving negative situations.
- Working to be more positive in their own interactions with and toward others.

Ask, **"Are there any changes you are willing to try before our next meeting?"** While discussing these ideas, you can add arrows to the worksheet to indicate planned changes. Talk them through how they may go about making this change.

"Next, let's think back to last week when we discussed calm strategy options. I would like you to continue to try calm strategies this week with the same documentation. Try them each day and note how your body and mind feel before trying them and then again how they feel after trying the strategy." Show them Appendix M – Calming Practice. *"What options would you especially like to try this week?"* (Reference Appendix J to get ideas.) Support students if they want to try something but don't know exactly how to try it out (e.g., they want to do mindful meditation but need access to an app. Provide them with an appropriate app such as "Smiling Mind" that can support them with mindful meditation (Smiling Mind, 2020).

Wrap-up

"Your homework for this next week is to consider how you can enhance your inner circle to feel more positive. You can plan to take the steps we discussed today. In addition, last week you tried out different coping practices. This week I want you to do this again and possibly try some new or different coping strategies. Document trying these practices throughout the week on the Calming Practice." (Appendix M.) **"Next week we will discuss coping strategies more in depth. Before you leave, please choose a breathing choice from Appendix F"** *(A or C).*

Session 10 Clinician Notes

Introduction/Assessment

As you open the discussion with the student regarding progress since your last meeting, focus on what it was like for them to break problems apart by considering what is within and what is outside of their control. Oftentimes, people with worry take on more stress than is necessary regarding situations, and their worry is not always necessarily something they have control over. You might use some mindfulness-based strategies to help the student consider how it felt to observe their thoughts in this way. Have students consider what they recognized within their body when they were feeling stressed and how that changed as they continued being aware of what they had control over and what they did not have control over. It is important that you not make the student feel bad for having any certain thoughts but instead help them to become knowledgeable in observing their thoughts and understanding that there may be times their thoughts relate to the worry that they are feeling and sometimes there are worries that come up that are outside of their control.

When sharing a personal example with a student to express how you observe your own thoughts and notice the impact on your body, recognize how the student responds and note if they can consider their own observations of their body's response to stress. If they are unable, that's ok. Instead, talk them through an example that may be most appropriate for them and that they could relate to so that when the time comes after your meeting, they can recognize and become aware of this feeling. Some examples that could be used to support connection may be:

- For someone who is an avid sports player: *"When I am up for a free throw and we are down by one with one minute left on the clock, I can notice my heart starting to race, my jaw clenches, and my thoughts are focused completely on what will happen within the next few seconds surrounding my shot."*
- For someone who is often concerned about friend issues: *"If a friend doesn't respond when I say hi to them, I might recognize my stomach start to hurt, my heart start to race, and my thoughts focus on why that friend might not have said hi to me."*
- For someone who often struggles with academic worries you may share: *"As a test is handed out, I notice my hands begin to sweat, my eyes starting to dart, and my leg begin to bounce. My thoughts are focused on the test and how I may be impacted by my performance."*

Whichever example is used, make sure to express the point of recognizing their thoughts and an awareness of what is happening within their body. Noting that often we are reactive and judgmental as to what is happening rather than just being aware so that we may also work to acknowledge and shift our attention to what is within our control. Remind them that this can be done by taking a deep breath to refocus.

Main Lesson

Next, support is provided to the student in understanding what they value. For younger students or those requiring more examples, first try to express what attributes you notice within them and see if they can come up with further traits that are important to them. For instance, you may share that you often notice them checking in on a friend when they look sad and share that a word that would describe this would be "caring." Then, if further explanation is needed, you might share characteristics that you yourself value and explain to the student why they are important to you. It doesn't necessarily matter what words are shared, as we all have our own ideas of what is most valuable to us as a person. However, likely the characteristics will be those that are often globally viewed as positive attributes. If the student were to state something that is not generally seen as a positive attribute (e.g., lying, saying hurtful things), question the child more with something like, "*Oh really, lying is something that you value? Explain that more to me so I can understand why that might be something you value?*" Be cautious to not show judgment toward their answer and instead work with them to understand why they answered in this way. It is possible they didn't understand the question, that they have had lying reinforced in their life in some way, or they may just be trying to see how you will respond. Regardless, continue to question their responses with interest and curiosity but ultimately work to see how the more negative attribute could be listed as a positive characteristic.

It's also important to note to the student(s) that what is important to them now will likely change. Our experiences, age, and friendships can alter how we view the world and what is most important. That is ok and expected. Right now our focus is on the current moment.

After working with the student on what behaviors they themselves value, you'll then ask the student to think about behaviors from others. While completing this portion, ask the student to think about someone who they enjoy being around, someone that energizes them and makes them feel happy. Ask them to then write down the qualities of this person that they believe is a positive influence on them. If they need help, ask the student for examples of what this person may do or say to them if they were having a bad day. Or ask them how this person greets them when they see them? You can further explain an example by stating that you really appreciate when you're talking to someone, and you recognize they are truly listening. When someone listens while you talk, it feels helpful and good to you. They then can write down whatever behaviors they identify in the middle box of the worksheet.

When asking the student to think about negative characteristics, have them consider a time when they felt bothered by something that someone else said or did. Just as you did with the positive situation, work through this example with the student by understanding how the behaviors of that person in that moment might be described. Support the student in knowing that these are behaviors that a person may display, it does not necessarily mean that this person always acts in this way. If the student still struggles, you can offer your own example of something that is a challenging behavior for you. It's important you are genuine when sharing this information, but also don't overshare to influence the student's further thoughts. For example, you might explain that if someone tells you they are going to do something but then don't follow through and actually do what they said, it really makes you feel bad. With this example in mind, you would share with the student that the word you'd write down would be "unreliable."

The circle diagram is meant to provide a visual to the table that starts this discussion on the impact of others. The middle circle signifies that they are the center and most important in their world. The people within the other circles can impact them as a person, but they can determine who is worthy to be close to them and who should be kept at a distance. Therefore, have the student first write down which people are closest to them in their life in the inner circle. Oftentimes this is going to be the family they live with and best friends. Next, the student is directed to write down which people are a part of their life but not necessarily close to them and write them in the outer circle. After that they can write down anyone else that feels significant to them but doesn't fall into either of the circles and place these names outside of all the circles. Whoever is on this diagram is completely up to the student. Once they feel like they have all the names written on the diagram, they will begin thinking about their influence on them as a person. Ask them to think about each person and how they make them feel. For this activity have the student become aware of their body and any signals they may get when they think of a certain name. As they do this, have them place a +, −, or both +/− next to the name. As this process is happening, wait to add discussion until they are finished unless they appear to need support.

Once the student is done marking each name with how they influence them, ask the student to consider if they missed documenting any people on the diagram and give them an opportunity to add names and the appropriate symbol if needed. Then, have the student look at their diagram and ask them to consider how they want to feel. You can use a brief visualization prompt by asking them to pause and consider how their body and mind would feel if they only allowed positive people into their inner circle. Discuss this idea and feeling with the student.

Ask the student to add arrows to show moving people in and out of circles with a goal to support their well-being. It's important to share with the student that when someone else makes us feel bad, that impacts our overall mood and can make us have more negative thoughts. Therefore, it's important to be aware of the people who surround us so that time can be focused on building relationships with positive influences.

Note: for this section, there is a chance that some of the people that the students identify as having more of a negative influence may be within the student's personal family circle and/or unchangeable in their relationship. In this case, support the student by acknowledging their concerns and talking about options that they may have to build their relationships with others that are positive and minimize time around those that are more negative in their influence. For instance, if their parents are often fighting and yelling at them, alternative options at home may be discussed such as coloring in the bedroom when parents are upset, calling a relative that makes them feel happy more often, or walking outside with a friend who is helpful (with parent permission).

Wrap-up

For homework, the student is expected to make one small change to influence themselves for the better. If the student needs clarification on this activity, offer that they could choose to spend less time with someone that often makes them feel badly, they may try to spend more time with someone that makes them feel good, or they may try to become more aware of others' influences on them by recognizing in the moment if someone is making them feel happy or badly. Ask them if they have an idea of what this one small change can be. Then, document their plan for the check in the next session.

In addition, provide the student with another Calming Practice (Appendix M) handout. Explain that you'd like them to continue trying out new practices this week and documenting how it goes in terms of changing their feelings.

Teacher and Guardian Summary

Hello, for our session this week, we were focused on what characteristics are important to us. We considered these characteristics while also thinking about the people that surround us. There was reflection on how the people around us influence our inner thoughts. We documented where we believe these people fall in their relationship to us (within our inner circle and someone we trust and share secrets with, within our outer circle and someone that's close but not someone that we'd share secrets with, or someone outside of our circle – we see them routinely but don't share a connection). After considering the characteristics that your child identified as important, we then discussed whether these people are helpful in building our positive characteristics or if they hinder our thoughts and make them more negative.

Homework

I gave a challenge to make one small change that can influence them for the better. Throughout this next week, help to generalize this learning by using the word "influence" when talking about the people with whom you surround yourself. Also, you might offer to share characteristics that are important to you with your child. In addition, your student was once again asked to continue their practice of coping strategies at least three times over the next week. We will explore coping options more thoroughly next week.

Work Cited

Smiling Mind. "Smiling Mind." *Smiling Mind*, 2020, www.smilingmind.com.au/.

11 Coping Strategies

Session 11 Outline

Focus

This chapter is all about calming/stress reduction practices. Students have a chance to practice three different types of calming strategies – mindful meditation is introduced with a progressive muscle relaxation; yoga is practiced through a tree pose; creativity is exercised through drawing, coloring, and writing; and gratitude is applied by considering three things of which the student is grateful.

Learning Targets

- Students will be able to explore different forms of stress reduction including mindfulness, movement, creativity, and gratitude.
- Students will be able to identify which form of stress reduction they see as most beneficial for themselves.

Materials Needed

- Group rules (if applicable).
- Pencil and paper for your notes.
- Pencil or pen for student.
- Appendix D – Weekly Assessment.
- Yoga mat (optional).
- Pillow or cushion for the floor (optional).
- Coloring book or coloring pages.
- Device to play music.
- Crayons/markers/colored pencils (optional).
- Appendix L – Calm Strategy Rating.

Introduction/Assessment

"It's nice to see you today. I am curious how your small change for the better went." Reference what they shared last time if they planned with you. Respond by listening to their response. If they were successful, congratulate them on their focus to make a positive change for themselves. If they were not successful or didn't try anything, ask them about a plan to try again or alter their original plan.

"I'm also wondering how using calming strategies went. Did you try anything new or different?" Pause, listen, and respond. "Please take a few minutes to complete the Weekly Assessment (Appendix D)."

DOI: 10.4324/9781003324782-11

Main Lesson

"Each week we have taken time to talk about something that can work as a coping strategy. Today we are going to spend the entire time together, practicing different types of relaxation methods. We are going to start our time with a mindful listening exercise. We will then get in a little bit of movement by doing a short yoga sequence. Next, we will listen to calming music while coloring, drawing, or writing (the student's choice). "Finally, we will end with you naming three things of which you are grateful. I am going to have you rate your experience with the Calm Strategy Rating" (Appendix L) so that we know what strategies seem to be most helpful for you. Let's get started."

"We will begin with a short, guided meditation practice. This practice is known as Progressive Muscle Relaxation" (Jacobson, 1987). "I am going to guide you through a process of noticing the different parts of your body by focusing your awareness and then tensing and relaxing your muscles. I invite you to get comfortable. You may choose to lay on the ground (offer a yoga mat if one is available), you may sit in a chair, or you may sit on the floor (offer a floor cushion if one is available). Now, I am going to have you listen to my voice and focus your awareness on your breath and body."

"Take a deep breath in through your nose and out through your mouth. You may close your eyes or gaze slightly downward at the floor. Take another deep breath in through your nose and out through your mouth.

Shift your attention to your feet …. As you focus on the sensations within your feet, take a deep breath in and squeeze your feet muscles together, squeezing, squeezing…. Release your muscles and breathe out through your mouth.

Next, move your attention toward your legs …. Consider what your legs do for you … take a deep breath in through your nose and tighten your leg muscles …. Include your calf and thighs both as you tighten, tighten …. then release your legs and breathe out through your mouth.

Now, move up to your stomach. Notice what you feel inside of your stomach…. Take a deep breath in and tighten your stomach muscles … tighten … tighten … Breathe out and release your stomach.

Focus on your shoulders. Become aware of whether they already seem to be tense or relaxed … breathe in through your nose and tighten your shoulders by bringing them up to your ears … tighten … tighten … now take a deep breath out and drop your shoulders down.

Move your awareness to your arms and hands… Recognize where you may hold any tightness… then take a deep breath in, holding, holding, squeeze your arm muscles by stiffening your arms and then squeezing your hands shut as if you were squeezing a lemon in your hands… squeezing… squeezing… relax your arms and hands as you breathe outward.

Now, become aware of all the smaller muscles inside of your face… tighten up each muscle…your nose should scrunch…your lips pursing…your eyebrows furrowed… then take a deep breath and release.

Finally, we are going to work through all the parts of your body. As I say the area, continue holding that part of your body until I ask you to release it. Start by taking a deep breath in… holding your breath and squeezing your feet… now your legs… then your stomach…and your shoulders… next your arms and hands… and lastly the muscles in your face… hold these muscles tense as you hold your breath… squeeze… now take a deep breath out through your mouth and release all these muscles at once.

Take one more deep breath in through your nose and out through your mouth. Begin to bring your awareness to the room. If your eyes have been closed, you may slowly open them."

"Pay attention to how your body feels right now … Also, notice your thoughts and whether you feel more aware of them. Please rate your perception of this experience as it relates to your body and mind on the Calm Strategy Rating (Appendix L), from tense and unsettled to calm and relaxed.

Now, we are going to transition to a movement activity. We will practice different variations of tree pose." Do the pose with the student as you provide the instructions.

"Begin by standing and taking a deep breath in and straightening your spine as if there is a string on top of your head pulling you toward the ceiling. Slowly breathe out and feel your feet grounded on the floor, balanced.

Next, breathe in and move your right foot up to your heel, as you breathe out focus on feeling balanced as you shift your weight to your left foot. Take another breath in and slowly move your foot up to a spot on your left leg that is comfortable. You might try your calf or your thigh. Be cautious to not rest your foot on your knee. If you are comfortable resting your right foot on your ankle that is just fine. Slowly breathe in through your nose and out through your mouth.

Take another deep breath in through your nose and raise both hands to the sky. As you breathe out, move your hands outward into the shape of a v.

Take three more slow deep inhales and exhales while in this position. It can be helpful to focus on something with your eyes to support you in your balance. Inhale... exhale... inhale..... exhale.... inhale... and on your next exhale slowly bring your arms to your sides and your right foot back onto the ground.

Take a deep breath in through your nose and out through your mouth. Bring your awareness to your right leg. As you breathe in deeply, shift your weight to your right foot and begin to bring your left foot up toward your right heel to rest on your right foot. As you feel more comfortable take a breath in and move your left foot up to rest on your calf or thigh of the right leg.

On your next in breath, slowly bring your hands up to the sky. As you take a breath out, shift your hands outward into a v type of position. Maintain this pose for three more deep breaths in through your nose and out through your mouth. Remember to focus your eyes on something that is steady to help you maintain your balance.

On your third breath out, slowly bring your hands back to your sides and your feet to the ground. Take another deep breath in through your nose and out through your mouth. Focus on how grounded your body feels at this moment."

"Notice what thoughts arose during that exercise as well as how it felt to move your body in that way. Considering your experience, complete your rating of this activity." Cue them to fill in the yoga section of the Calm Strategy Rating – Appendix L.

"We are now going to move into an activity that touches more on creativity. You have the option to utilize coloring pages, blank sheets of papers, or a notebook so that you may color, draw, or write during this time." Refer them to these items in your space. "I will turn on a timer for five minutes and will play calming music during this time." Play any calm music found through an internet search or music readily available in your room. "Let's get started."

Start a timer for five minutes. Allow the student to choose an option. Throughout the five minutes, state reminders such as, "Notice how your writing utensil feels on the paper. Recognize how your body is responding to creating in this way. How is your mood?" All these questions are meant as rhetorical questions and not necessarily anything that is expected to be answered. Therefore, you may remind students that you are asking these questions to get them thinking but not necessarily to hear an answer. After five minutes, ask them, "finish up what you are doing. I would now like you to rate this experience and how it felt for your mind and body." Guide them in responding to the questions under creativity.

"Now, before you leave, I want you to say or write three things that you are grateful for in your life. You may say something regarding yourself as a person, something that you are thankful to have that supports your life, a person that is especially helpful, or any other thing that makes you feel grateful as you consider its impact on you and your life. I am going to give you a minute to think about what you'd like to acknowledge." Pause and wait a minute. "Now, please share three things

that make you feel grateful." Pause and wait until all three things are noted. "Now, go ahead and rate your experience of considering things of which you're grateful. Consider this impact on your mind... and body" (referencing Appendix L).

Wrap-up

"**As we finalize our time together, my hope is that both your body and mind are feeling calmer. I would like you to shift your awareness to the Calm Strategy Rating (Appendix L). Notice which category most stands out. Which seemed to be most beneficial to your mind and your body. If multiple areas stand out, consider what you feel was best for you, and what you most enjoyed doing today. Before you leave, write your favorite activity on your Calm Strategy Rating worksheet with a star next to that activity. You are going to leave this worksheet with me. Over the next week, I am going to challenge you once again to practice a calming strategy at least three times and document how this went for you.**" (Hand them Appendix M – Calming Practice). "**Think about ways in which you can be more engaged in this type of coping and bring this completed sheet back with you next week.**"

Session 11 Clinician Notes

Introduction/Assessment

When asking the student(s) about how their homework for changes to relationships went the last week, be prepared for a successful completion of this activity, an unsuccessful attempt, or not trying at all. Note that if you are addressing this in a group, you may want to keep a student who was unsuccessful afterward to identify what is most needed so that you can have a more individualized and confidential discussion. You may also choose to offer to all students in a group the opportunity to write down their thoughts on how it went rather than speak in front of others.

- Successful attempt: ask the student more about how it felt to attempt this change. Check in with them about whether feelings of worry came up for them and if so, ask them how they handled that worry. Acknowledge to them that worry is an expected emotion in this situation as they are attempting to make a change in the way they've known things. Changes can be scary, even if we anticipate they are for the best.
- Unsuccessful attempt: work to understand how they attempted the change. Learn about what they did, what support they had available to them, and what went wrong. Support them in analyzing what needs to change for next time. It may mean creating a new goal or it might require a different type of plan in how to carry out the change. Help the student(s) in identifying what is needed and plan together.
- No attempt: ask the student(s) to share with you about what made it challenging to attempt to follow through with the plan. Some things that may get in the way are time, forgetting, avoiding the change, or feeling as though the change is too overwhelming. Remind them that you will be checking in again next week and want to make sure that we create a plan that can be followed through with this time. Support them in considering what may need to change to follow through with the plan. Alter their goal if that feels more appropriate. Also make sure to identify supports they have that can help in making this change feel less scary.

Check in regarding how trying coping strategies went for the student(s) and see if they tried anything new. As the student(s) complete the assessment sheet, offer support with any questions that arise.

Main Lesson

Make sure that for this lesson you have all materials out and ready so that there is minimal transition time between trying each of the coping strategies. The goal of this session is for the student(s) to try a variety of calming strategies even if they are not completely comfortable with them. If a student expresses a feeling of worry or dislike in an activity, encourage them that it will be short lived and done in a safe setting. However, also be especially vigilant of any of these practices bringing up past trauma. If a student appears visibly distressed during any of the activities, calmly have them stop and offer an alternative option for them while the rest of the group finishes that exercise. Before starting the next activity, check in with them and see if they are comfortable returning and trying something else. If they are, welcome them back to the group. If not, offer them returning to their class or another quiet space and then check in with them later.

For students who need alternative options, you may ask them what feels most comfortable for them to try. It would be ideal if one of the strategies you are teaching were of interest to them. However, if the strategies aren't of interest to them at all, look at options that include less calm and more movement and distracted thinking. You might offer an opportunity to walk outside, complete a puzzle, or have them fidget with something like putty, magnets, or water beads.

As they complete ratings, offer to support them with any questions that come up regarding their feeling of calm. If further examples or explanation are needed for the ratings, ask them what they believe it feels like to feel calm within their body. Then also ask what it feels like to feel calm within their mind. Have them think about that feeling as if it were the rating from tense to calm and have them consider how their body and mind felt after each exercise in comparison to that idea.

- Progressive muscle relaxation – while reading the script to the student, ensure that it is read in a calm and gentle tone. Take time while having them focus on each different part of the body. Choose your position in the room so that the student(s) don't feel like they are being watched or judged throughout this process. A supportive seat may be in the corner of the room where you yourself are also gazing downward. For students who are new to this exercise, explain that *"Paying attention to the body in this way can be challenging as it slows down our thinking and focuses our awareness. However, doing this helps to train the mind to become more aware and accepting of thoughts that come up. It can also allow us to be more ok with not responding to these thoughts."*
- Yoga/tree pose – while working through this practice, offer your own variations of tree pose for the students as feels appropriate. The important piece is working to pay attention to the movements of the body, practicing balance, and slightly challenging the body. Pay attention to the student(s) and recognize if they seem to be getting too challenged by movements they are making and gently re-direct them to try something less challenging. It can be common to struggle with balance. Remind them to focus on something in front of them that is not moving. It can also be offered that they do not need to move their foot up their leg and can instead use the opposing foot like a kickstand and lean it on the active foot. For individuals wanting more of a challenge with their arms, offer alternatives like bringing their hands together and placing them next to their chest. Another option is to sway their hands toward one side, slightly bending their elbows. Continue to remind the student(s) to pay attention to your words, their body movement, and their breath.
- Creativity exercise – have a small journal, coloring books, coloring pages, and plain paper sitting out for the students to choose from for this activity. In addition, offer different types of writing utensils including crayons, markers, pencils, pens, or colored pencils. Allow the students to use their own creativity to drive this activity. If prompts are needed for individual students to get them started, offer, *"draw or share about something that makes you happy."* For the calming music, there are many options available through internet searches. Try to stick with music that has calming sounds but does not include words so that students are less likely to get distracted.
- Gratitude exercise (three things) – offer again the resources used in the creativity exercise. Students can either write out three things that they are grateful for, or they can share out loud. Calming music can be on while the students think about what they are grateful for in life. Start this activity with examples so that sharing can be modeled in a specific way. For instance, *"I am grateful for the sound of my child's laughter as it reminds me that even small things can make us feel happy."*

You can also share an example of something you are grateful for that makes your life feel easier such as, "*I am grateful to have my garage connected to my house so that I don't have to freeze to warm up my car on my way in to work each day.*" Another example could be something about yourself as a person like, "*I am thankful for my strong legs that allow me to run and release the stress I feel within my body.*" Praise specific components of what students share. You may also ask further if you feel their example is too broad, "*What is it that you love most about ….*"

Wrap-up

As the student considers their ratings of each activity, if some of the strategies come out with similar ratings, encourage them to think about what they liked about the exercise and what they preferred to use most or can see themselves using again. Support the student with any questions that arise as they complete their assessment sheet and thank them for being open to trying new things with you during this session. You may also want to remind them if they are needing to make any changes within their relationships that weren't completed from last week. In addition, have them continue to complete the Calm Strategy Rating (Appendix M) at least three times over the next week.

Teacher and Guardian Summary

As you are aware, we've been spending a lot of time focusing on strategies to support stress and worry. This week we focused most of our time on trying out different types of calming techniques. Our time began together with a guided breathing practice where I guided your student in a practice to tighten and relax different parts of their body in sync with their breath. Next, they practiced balance and yoga through tree pose. After yoga, there was a creative choice of writing, coloring, or drawing while listening to mindful music. We finished by reflecting on our gratitude and naming three things of which we are thankful.

Homework

Please ask your student about their experience in trying these calming practices. Share with your student your favorite type of calm strategy as well. Check in with them regarding their plan for practicing. If you are willing, offer to practice with them.

Work Cited

Jacobson, E. (1987). Progressive relaxation. *The American Journal of Psychology, 100*(3/4), 522–537.

12 Student Plan

Session 8 Outline

Focus

The focus of this chapter is to review all of the learning that has taken place up until this point and put it together into a student plan. The goal for the plan is to remind the student of useful strategies when they are feeling stressed. The plan is also expected to support in generalization of learning and increasing positive supports which is done by sharing the plan with people close to the student including teachers and guardians.

Learning Targets

- Students will identify a plan to support them in feeling calm.
- Students will determine people who will be supportive in their calm plan.

Materials Needed

- Group rules (If applicable).
- Pencil and paper for your notes.
- Pencil or pen for student.
- Student notes/prior ratings from previous weeks.
- Large sheet of paper/whiteboard – something to write on for all to see.
- Student Worry Plan – Appendix N.
- Bag of small candy or trinkets (optional).
- Any short game (optional).

Introduction/Assessment

"How has your week been?" Pause, listen, and respond. **"Have you had a chance to practice some of the calming strategies? Let's see your Calming Practice Worksheet** (Appendix M)." Review their practices with them and ask questions about how it felt for them, what they most appreciated as a calming exercise, and when they found these strategies to be most useful (what was happening). Next, if the student needed to alter their plan for a change related to themselves and their relationships, ask the student about how this plan worked. "Please take a minute to complete the Weekly Assessment (Appendix D)."

Main Lesson

"This is our eighth time meeting. We've talked a lot about strategies that can help you when you are feeling anxious. Today we are going to create a plan to help keep everyone aware of what to look for when you start feeling worried as well as what can help. Before we get started working on the plan, let's reflect on what we've discussed during all of our weeks together." Get out whatever you are writing on and display it so that if you are working with a group, the whole group can see.

DOI: 10.4324/9781003324782-12

If you'd like to reward sharing out lessons learned, have a small bag of candy or trinkets ready and each time a student shares out, throw them a piece of candy or a trinket. Once you are done, you can let all students have the rest of the candy or divide out trinkets.

Review Game

"Alright, what can you remember from our time together?" To encourage sharing out, remind them that they will earn a piece of candy or trinket for sharing. Work to ensure that they touch on each of the following. If they don't, give them a hint to help them remember. While discussion occurs, add their idea on the board/paper being used to document thoughts.

- Deep breathing options (children: 4-7-8, finger breathing, and belly breathing); (adolescents: 4-7-8 breathing, 5-4-3-2-1, and shoulder breathing)
  - Hint: we learned about something that helps to calm your body.
- Body clues – where we notice the feeling of worry within our body.
  - Hint: what kind of signs can tell us that we are feeling worried?
- An awareness of different kinds of emotions:
  - Hint:
    - Children: we learned a lot about … (show your face making different gestures).
    - Adolescents: we talked a lot about how we may feel in different kinds of situations. How we feel might also be called … (the word you are looking for is – *emotions*).
- Changing/reframing thoughts – worst-case scenario, evidence against worst case scenario, best case scenario, and most likely scenario.
  - Hint: when you notice you are getting stuck in worst case/negative thinking, you can do this instead.
- Considering the possible options to work through a problem:
  - Hint: is there only one way to solve a problem? … What did we think about when considering alternative ways to solve a problem?
- What is in our control (Play-Doh) and what is outside of our control (rock)?
  - Hint: Play-Doh and rock – what did we say those stand for?
- Relationships that support positive thinking:
  - Hint: people we want to be around and are helpful to us support what kind of thinking?
- Relationships that create negative thinking:
  - Hint: people we're around but are not helpful to our thinking can create what type of thinking?
- Coping and stress reduction practices – yoga, mindful breathing, drawing, writing, gratitude, connection, etc.
  - Hint: strategies that can be used to make us feel more calm.

Student Worry Plan (Appendix N)

"Thinking about all that we have learned, you are going to create a worry plan that you can use as a reminder of what can be tried when you are feeling worried. This plan will also be helpful for us to share with your guardians and teachers so that they know how best to support you if you begin to feel anxious." Show them the Student Worry Plan (Appendix N). **"As we go through this plan, I am going to leave what we've written down about our learnings on this paper/board. That way**

if you get stuck, we can look back and remember what we've already learned and what may be most helpful to add in your plan."

- I can recognize I am starting to feel worried by paying attention to my body and mind.

  - ○ **"Let's first consider, I can recognize I am starting to feel worried by paying attention to my body and mind … What do you recognize as feelings that come up for you in your body? Where do you experience the worry?"** Pause and allow them to write or you write for them. **"What do you recognize happens in your mind? What is going on with your thoughts?."** Pause and allow them to write or you write for them.

- When I am worried, others may recognize me doing this …

  - ○ **"Now… When I am worried, others may recognize me doing this … How can others recognize you are worried? What clues does your body give? How might you act differently?."** Pause and allow them to write or you write for them.

- When I am feeling worried, the following things can help:

  - ○ **"When you are feeling worried, which of the strategies listed is most helpful for you? You are welcome to circle as many of these items as you'd like."** Read aloud each item as they follow along. Pause and allow them to circle if they'd prefer, after each word is read. **"You can also add anything that you would like to use but is not listed."**

- If the strategies I try on my own don't work, these people can help me when I am feeling anxious …

  - ○ **"If once you try those strategies, they don't work, who are some people that can help you?."** Encourage adults to be mentioned in addition to friends. Also encourage someone at school as well as in the home to be written down.

- This person can help by …

  - ○ **"How can that person be helpful?"** Read options with them, then pause, and allow them to circle and think of anything to add.

- It is not helpful when someone …

  - ○ **"What should be known for that person to NOT do if you are feeling anxious?"** Prompt them to think about what kinds of things someone may say or do that may make them more worried or feel frustrated.

- I will know I am feeling better by paying attention to my body and mind.

  - ○ **"Once you are feeling calm, how does your mind feel; how does your body feel? Let's write that down so that we can know when you might be ready to rejoin with whatever has been happening at school or at home."** Pause and support the student with ideas from what you've learned about them. You may also help in writing for the student if that support is needed.

"Now that you are finished with your plan, let's think about who should have a copy of your plan?" Pause and listen. If they don't name their guardian or a teacher, encourage that they are someone with whom you'd like to share this plan. Ask the student about their preference in who should share the plan. **"Would you like to be the one to share a copy of the plan to each of these individuals? Or would you prefer that I share the plan with them?"** Honor whatever they come up with as a response. **"Now that we have a plan for who will be given a copy, where do you think a good place would be for you to keep this plan as a reminder for yourself when you begin feeling anxious?"** Pause, listen, and support with ideas. **"Great, it's a good idea to have it somewhere that can be easily accessed because when our mind is feeling stressed, we sometimes can have a hard time remembering skills that have been learned for how to help calm down. If you want another copy of this sheet, I could make a second one so that you have it at both school and at home."** Honor their thoughts and if they decline, offer that if they change their mind, you can always make another copy for them later.

If there is enough time left over, offer to play a short game with them. If you don't have a game available, you could offer to play tic-tac-toe or go out on a short walk for fresh air together. If there isn't enough time, go to the wrap-up portion.

Wrap-up

"You have worked so hard during our time together to become more aware of your thoughts, emotions, and responses. As we discussed, please take your Worry Plan with you." If appropriate based on the plan you created, have them also take the worry plans for the other people that are supporting them. Make sure that you have a copy for yourself. **"Next week I would like to hear about the use of this plan. I also want you to know that next week is our last week working through these strategies together. Think about how you feel things have been going as compared to when we first started meeting and we can talk about next steps when we talk next week."**

Week 8 Clinician Notes

Introduction/Assessment

As you check in about how the week has been, pay specific attention to the calming strategies that the student(s) have tried. In reviewing their Calming Practice worksheet (Appendix M), ask them their thoughts about what type of strategy seemed to work best. Note if they seemed to prefer one certain type of practice or if they tried a variety. If they only did one certain type of practice, ask them what got in the way of them trying something different. If they tried multiple practices, ask them about which type was their favorite.

If a student needed to alter their plan for a relationship, check in and ask about how this strategy went for them. Ask questions about what a challenge was and what made them feel successful. Inquire about how they felt after making this change. Follow where the conversation leads. Then support the student with any questions that arise during the Weekly Assessment (Appendix D).

Main Lesson

Review Game

If using candy for this lesson, check with teacher/guardians regarding any food allergies/sensitivities ahead of time. You could expand upon the knowledge check-in by creating a game such as fill in the blank, jeopardy, or charades. To determine what your student(s) would most respond to, consider if they seem to be more motivated by a lot of action and games or if they do best by talking through the lesson. You might also offer students to share what week they found to be most helpful to them.

Support the student(s) in reviewing skill gaps and reminding them about the different strategies learned if they struggle to recall information. Provide positive feedback for accurate statements and expand upon learning to ask for examples of the strategies being used.

Student Worry Plan (Appendix N)

As you complete the Student Worry Plan (Appendix D) with the student, offer small reminders for each section to support them in thinking through each response. Some tips that can be used are below.

- I can recognize I am starting to feel worried by paying attention to my body and mind.

  - *"I've noticed that you especially expressed* (state name of body region) *being bothered by your worry."*
  - *"You've also shared that your mind…"* (e.g., often thinks about how other people will respond negatively, such as them laughing at you).

- When I am worried, others may recognize me doing this …

  o *"I've recognized that when you are worried you tend to … (e.g., twirl your hair), what is something you notice you do that your teacher/parent could recognize as a sign that you could benefit from additional support because you're feeling anxious?"*

- When I am feeling worried, the following things can help:

  o *"When you are feeling worried, which of the strategies listed is most helpful for you? You are welcome to circle as many of these items as you'd like"* (read aloud each item as they follow along. Pause and allow them to circle if they'd prefer, after each word is read). *"You can also add any additional strategies."*

- If the strategies I try on my own don't work, these people can help me when I am feeling worried …

  o *"Who are the people that are most supportive and helpful in a positive way of your worry? Let's think back to the people in your inner circle that had a positive sign next to them."*

- This person can help by …

  o *"What is helpful from others when you are feeling anxious? Is it something they say or do that can be helpful?"* (e.g., letting me sit by myself for a while, or talking through the situation with me to help me see the most likely scenario vs. the worst-case scenario).

- It is not helpful when someone …

  o *"What are some of those characteristics that others may display that are bothersome to you, and would not be helpful?"* (e.g., asking too many questions, trying to get me to do something creative).

- I will know I am feeling better by paying attention to my body and mind.

  o *"Remember when we did the relaxation practices last week? Think about how your body and mind felt then … Now let's try to capture those feelings into words and write them down"* (e.g., still, relaxed, and focused).

Reference back to worksheets that they had completed in previous weeks and remind them of what came up for them, e.g., *"You noted on the Calming Strategy Rating that yoga seemed to make the most improvement in your mind and body, is that something that can be part of your coping strategy? You had your mom listed as someone that is helpful on your Positive/Negative Influences and Relationships worksheet, maybe she would be a good person to note as being able to help."*

As you talk with the student about where they will keep their worksheet, remind them to also think about what kind of cue (e.g., my heart starts to race and I can't focus) will remind them to look at the sheet and think logically through the calming steps. It's important to consider these types of things to help ensure the work you've been doing together can be generalized. In addition to the student having a plan for keeping their own worksheet, this chapter encourages the student to also share a worksheet with people that can support them. There is an option for you to share the sheet for the student or for the student to share it themselves. Students who are especially quiet or reserved may feel anxious about giving this plan to someone else. In that case, share the plan with the adults they name and ask that the person share with the student in some way that they got the plan. The trusted adult may choose to talk through the plan with the student or they may say, *"I received your Student Worry Plan and I want you to know I've looked it over and feel ready to help if you need me. Please reach out if you ever need more help."* If the student feels comfortable and would like to give the plan to the adults named, talk them through what that will look like. Ask questions like, *"When would be a good time for you to give them this plan?"* and have them consider how many others might be around along with the person's potential for distractability at any certain time. Also ask, *"What will you say to them about the plan?"* explain that they might share that this is something that can help them when they are worried and they'd like the adult to have a copy so that they know how to help them if needed.

If there is enough time remaining in the session, follow the student's lead with what they may want to do with the remaining time together. Consider the short games listed as options or walking outside while talking about anything they want. Ask them about how life is going – what is going well, what is not going so well.

Wrap-up

As you wrap up the session, make sure to remind the student of the plan for the Student Worry Plan – where they will keep their copy and how others will be notified. To support the student with reflecting throughout the next week, you might encourage that they use a journal to keep track of how often they use the plan as well as what they've most appreciated through this time together.

Teacher and Guardian Summary

Today, during our time together, we reviewed what we have learned over the past few weeks. We then compiled our learning together into a Student Worry Plan that includes signs of when your student is feeling worried as well as what can help them with these feelings. I am attaching the plan we created together to this email OR – your student will be sharing this plan with you.

Homework

It would be helpful if you can work with your student to talk with them about their worry plan and assure them that you will be supportive of them when they need you. You might also ask your student to share their thoughts about the plan and where they will keep it so that they have it when they need.

13 Completion/Next Steps

Session 9 Outline

Focus

The focus of this chapter is to gather data to understand how these last nine weeks have supported the student's level of anxiety and awareness of coping strategies. There is also a final practice in supporting the student in feeling prepared to use these strategies independently.

Learning Targets

- Students will identify what they continue to need in order to be successful in coping with their worry.

Materials Needed

- Pencil and paper.
- Pencil or pen for student.
- Appendix C – Pre/Post Test.
- Appendix D – Weekly Assessment.
- Markers.

Introduction/Assessment

"How did using the Student Worry Plan go?" Pause, listen, and respond. **"Did you need to use it at all over the last week? Are there any changes you'd like to see made?"** If so, offer to support them in creating an updated form. **"Know that this is something that can be changed whenever you need. It's important that it is true to what can be most helpful for you."**

"This is our last week together. You might remember that when we started you completed an assessment, I am going to have you complete that assessment again so that I can understand how our time together has supported you." Give them Appendix C – Pre-Post Test. Read the questions aloud and support them with any questions. Next, hand them Appendix D – Weekly Assessment and say, **"This is your last time also taking this assessment."** Read the questions aloud and support them with any of their own questions.

Once the students(s) is/are complete with their assessments, ask the following questions and write down their answers for your notes.

- **"What do you feel has gone well during our time together?"**
- **"What did you not like about the past 9 weeks?"**

DOI: 10.4324/9781003324782-13

- **"How do you feel about us ending our time together?"**
- **"What supports will you use to help you continue to calm your worry?"**

*If you are in a group, you can offer to students that they can write their answers to these questions down if they'd prefer not to share them aloud.

Main Lesson

"For our last day together, I thought we'd plan a game and then end with a calming option of your choice." Feel free to choose with the student options below or offer to do something else together that they enjoy.

- Jenga (before pulling out a Jenga piece, the person whose turn it is needs to ask the person to their right a question. Reverse the order after everyone in the group has a chance).
- Kerplunk (similar to Jenga, before pulling out a stick, the person whose turn it is needs to ask the person to their right a question. Reverse the order after everyone in the group has a chance).
- Building together with magna tiles or Legos (talk while you work and build, ask the student questions about themselves and encourage them to ask questions to you).
- Drawing or coloring together (talk while you create, ask the student questions about themselves and encourage them to ask questions to you).
- Go for a walk outside and talk about life as you walk.
- Shoot hoops together and each time someone makes a basket, they share something about themselves that the others may not know.

Once you have about ten minutes left of your session time together, wrap up the activity. Ask the student(s), **"I would like us to spend one more time doing a calming activity of your choice together. What would you most like to do?"** Below are possible options.

- Mindful meditation – *"Find a comfortable seated position … Take a deep breath in through your nose and out through your mouth … In through your nose, and out through your mouth … As you begin to relax, you may close your eyes or gaze downward … Notice how it feels to pay attention to your breathing in this way … Become aware of the breath coming in through your nose, through your chest, and down to fill your stomach. Then back up and out through your mouth … As you continue breathing focus your attention on your breath and your body … When thoughts come up, acknowledge them and let them go … You may recognize different sounds, smells, and feelings … With this new awareness, be open and continue your focus on the breath … Breathing in and out … Breathing in and out … (pause quietly counting to yourself to 10) … on your next in breath, you may slowly begin to bring your focus to the room and open your eyes."*
- Yoga – *"Let's go through a seated chair pose. Begin by sitting on your chair with your bottom close to the middle or edge of the seat. Situate your sitting so that you feel stable and centered on the chair. Take a deep breath in and straighten your spine as if there is a piece of string tied to the top of your head pulling upward …Breathe out …On your next in breath, bring your left arm up and put your right arm down to your side. Breathe out and stretch your left fingers toward the right side of the room, bending your neck lightly … On your next in breath, bring your right arm up and put your left arm down to your side. Breathe out and stretch your right fingers toward the left side of the room, bending your neck lightly … Breathe in and take both arms up straight toward the ceiling … breathe out and bend your hands toward the floor … Stay in this position and take a deep breath in through your nose … as you breathe out slowly with your mouth come back up to seated position."*
- Creativity – have a piece of paper and markers ready. *"How about we draw a picture of our favorite memory."* Take about five minutes to do this and then have everyone share out about what was drawn. Calm music can be playing in the background.
- Gratitude – have paper and writing utensil options ready. *"We are going to write a letter to someone for whom we are grateful. Take a moment to think about who this person is and why you are grateful they are a part of your life. Once you are ready, you can start writing."* Allow five minutes and then ask them if they'd like to give this letter to the person. You can provide options of support if needed for delivery.

Once finished, **"How did this activity feel for you? … Is it something you'd try again?"** Listen and take mental note of responses. **"Remember, there are many different ways that you can work through feelings of stress and worry, we've just touched on some of those practices. Although many people use calming practices when they are feeling worried or stressed, they can be most useful if they are part of a common practice in your everyday life."**

Wrap-up

"As we end our time together, I want you to think about how you will continue to utilize the practices that we've learned together. How might you continue to incorporate these practices into your week?" (Listen) **"Do you have an idea for how you can help yourself to be accountable to sticking with your plan?"** Listen and provide feedback. **"I am thankful we had this time to get to know each other better. Please remember that although this** (group/one-on-one) **time has ended, if something comes up, you can always reach out to me by …"** Share with them the best way to make contact with you moving forward. **"I am proud of you and your growth. I hope you are proud of yourself too."**

Session 9 Clinician Notes

Introduction/Assessment

When checking in about how use of the Student Worry Plan (Appendix N) has gone for the student, gather specific information about what was helpful or not-so-helpful so that necessary changes can be made. It may be particularly helpful if feedback could be gathered from the teacher and guardian ahead of this session.

Be ready to write down answers to the additional questions that are asked of the student(s). The information gathered from them today should be used to then create a plan for them moving forward. After the assessment, the data will be reviewed to determine next steps to share with the guardian, teacher, and student. Use the appropriate bullet points below to determine possibilities for what can happen next.

- Data shows an improvement in skills.
  - Set up plan for student to be able to reach out to you if something comes up and they recognize they need your support.
  - Remind them to continue to reference their Student Worry Plan.
- Data remains similar across time.
  - Consider an additional layer of support for the student based on needs and interest.
    - Continuation of regular meetings with you.
    - Check-ins/skill teaching/regulation support – with another trusted adult.
- Data shows a decline in skills.
  - Work with the team (teacher, guardian, any other staff, or outside providers supporting the student) to determine what may be most helpful. Consider what approaches the student was responsive toward and those that they resisted.
    - Individualized meetings with another trusted adult.
    - Team discussion around individualized support options for the student.

Main Lesson

The point of the game is to do a final check in with the student(s) regarding their feelings and also to celebrate all of their hard work over the last few weeks. Additional options for games can be utilized if you are able to tie them into questions related to emotions or general check-in questions. When deciding on a game, you might offer the student two options from which they can choose to reduce choices.

As you move on to the calming activity, allow the student to choose. Other options that have been discussed in previous meetings include going for a walk, coloring with calming music, a deep breathing strategy, and free journaling with music. Also note that though there are examples for mindful meditation, yoga, creativity, and gratitude, the examples that are given do not need to be used. If you have an alternative strategy that can fall under one of these categories, it is ok to use that strategy instead.

While checking in with the student(s) regarding how they felt about the calming exercise, support them in considering their mind and body by asking reflection questions related to how these areas felt. This allows for awareness of what is going on within them. Asking questions in this way can also help to prompt them to be more aware of their body in future calming activities.

Students are asked to consider how they can continue to utilize these practices on a regular basis. It's important to support the student(s) with planning so that you can help them in thinking through when is the best time of the day to practice this strategy, how many days a week will work for them, and who else needs to be involved with this plan to support with accountability of follow through. If the student buys into planning and is a part of creating it with you, they are more likely to follow the plan because there is self-motivation.

Wrap-up

While discussing next steps, talk through specific ways that the student can continue a connection with you. Make sure that the student agrees to whatever plan is created in moving forward. Touch on: how the student can reach you, how they would like to have future check-ins and if continued meetings are going to happen.

Teacher/Guardian Summary

Today was our last meeting together. During our time today, we reviewed some information that has been learned and we also checked in about how feelings related to worry may have changed since we started meeting. Based on that data ... (use one of the following).

- If data shows an improvement in skills:
  - ... your child is showing an improvement from when we first began talking. I've specifically noticed they seem to be doing well with_____. Based on this information and discussions with your child, I would like to recommend that your student continue to utilize their Student Worry Plan and regular coping strategies. I've also talked with your student about how I can be reached if something were to come up for them from which they'd like my support.

- If data remains similar across time:
  - ... it appears that there hasn't been much change in skills since we first began talking. I did notice that they do well with _____ but that they continue to struggle with _____ . I would like to continue supporting your student. Some options we could consider are continuation of regular meetings with me or having them start meeting with another trusted adult at school (*you might include that person's title and how they can support differently*). Would there be a time we can talk further regarding your thoughts?

- If data shows a decline in skills:

  - ... it appears that there has actually been a decline in skills since we first began talking. I did notice that they do well with _____ but that they continue to struggle with _____ . I would like to continue supporting your student. Some options we could consider are continuation of regular meetings with me or having them start meeting with another trusted adult at school (*you might include that person's title and how they can support differently*), and/or a school team discussion that includes (_____ – *note anyone on your school student services team that would be a part of this discussion*). Would there be a time we can talk further regarding your thoughts?

Thank you for your continued support of your student. Please do not hesitate to reach out to me if any questions or concerns arise. I can be reached by e-mail at _____ and by phone at _____. Thank you and take care.

14 Continued Support for the Classroom

This section includes mini lessons for classroom teachers. The lessons could be used to provide additional support for a student or students who have been supported with the 9-week sessions in chapters 5–13, they could be used independently, or the lessons could be used as a whole class learning strategy. The lessons are intended to enhance emotional awareness and increase coping strategies. In addition to strategies, optional accommodations for use with students with anxiety are provided and example goals for students with individualized education plans are given. The following are summarized throughout this chapter:

- Emotions Check-in.
- Calm Space.
- Daily Mindfulness.
- Short Mindful Moments.
- Deep Breathing Graphics.
- Accommodations.
- Individualized Education Plan Goals.

DOI: 10.4324/9781003324782-14

Emotions Check-in

What It Is

- Quick and confidential check-in with students to see how they are feeling.
  - The check-in allows an understanding of how the class is feeling overall.
  - The check-in helps teachers to understand which students may be especially struggling so that they can provide them with additional time and support.

How It Looks

Emotion check-ins can be completed in many different ways, the following are some potential strategies for the classroom:

- Hard copy shared by all students.
  - Have a list of five different options of feelings – this can be on a whiteboard, a smartboard, or a large sheet of paper. The chart should look like that in *Figure 14.1*.
  - Have students write their names on the sticky side of a post-it note and then stick the note next to how they are feeling so that the blank side is what is seen. Say to students, *"First write your name on the sticky side of the post-it note. Then, take a deep breath and focus on what is happening within your body … and mind … Consider how you are feeling today – wonderful, happy, okay, a bit down, or really upset* (say this while pointing to each section). *Then place your post-it note next to the area that most accurately shows how you are feeling now."*
  - Next, *"Let's all look at what we notice from our check ins* (promote discussion of their reflection) – (e.g., if a few students chose a bit down or really upset, the question could be asked, "Are a couple of classmates feeling low? – how could we support these friends?). *Take a moment to think about whether your feelings changed from yesterday or stayed the same* (pause). *Now, thinking about how you are feeling, I want you to identify how you were feeling and think about what you want to do to help keep yourself feeling well, or what you may need to do to better help yourself to focus today. Would anyone want to share their ideas?"* (Pause and call on a few students who have thoughts on coping strategies to share).
- Emotion check-in handout/virtual completion.
  - Handout the emotion check-in for students to complete independently (*Figure 14.1*) (*Note: a hard copy can be made like that in *Figure 14.1*, or the questions can be asked on an electronic form that collects student name so that appropriate support can be provided when necessary).
  - Each day ask, *"Think about how you are feeling and mark that box. Then, write down a strategy you can use to either help keep yourself focused or to get your body to feel calm and focused for the day."* On Tuesdays, Wednesdays, Thursdays, and Fridays, also ask the students to reflect on the prior days that week and consider how their feelings have changed or stayed the same.

Notes of Caution

- Do not call out anyone that is feeling down in front of the classroom, find a private time to talk with them about their feelings.
- Do not punish the class or speak negatively about them feeling anything other than happy. If that occurs, it is best to simply acknowledge that's how everyone is feeling and then talk about what might help to boost the class mood.

Benefit

Emotion check-ins allow for an opportunity to share feelings and reflect. In the classroom, having all students participate in a personal reflection of their feelings allows for teacher awareness and peer

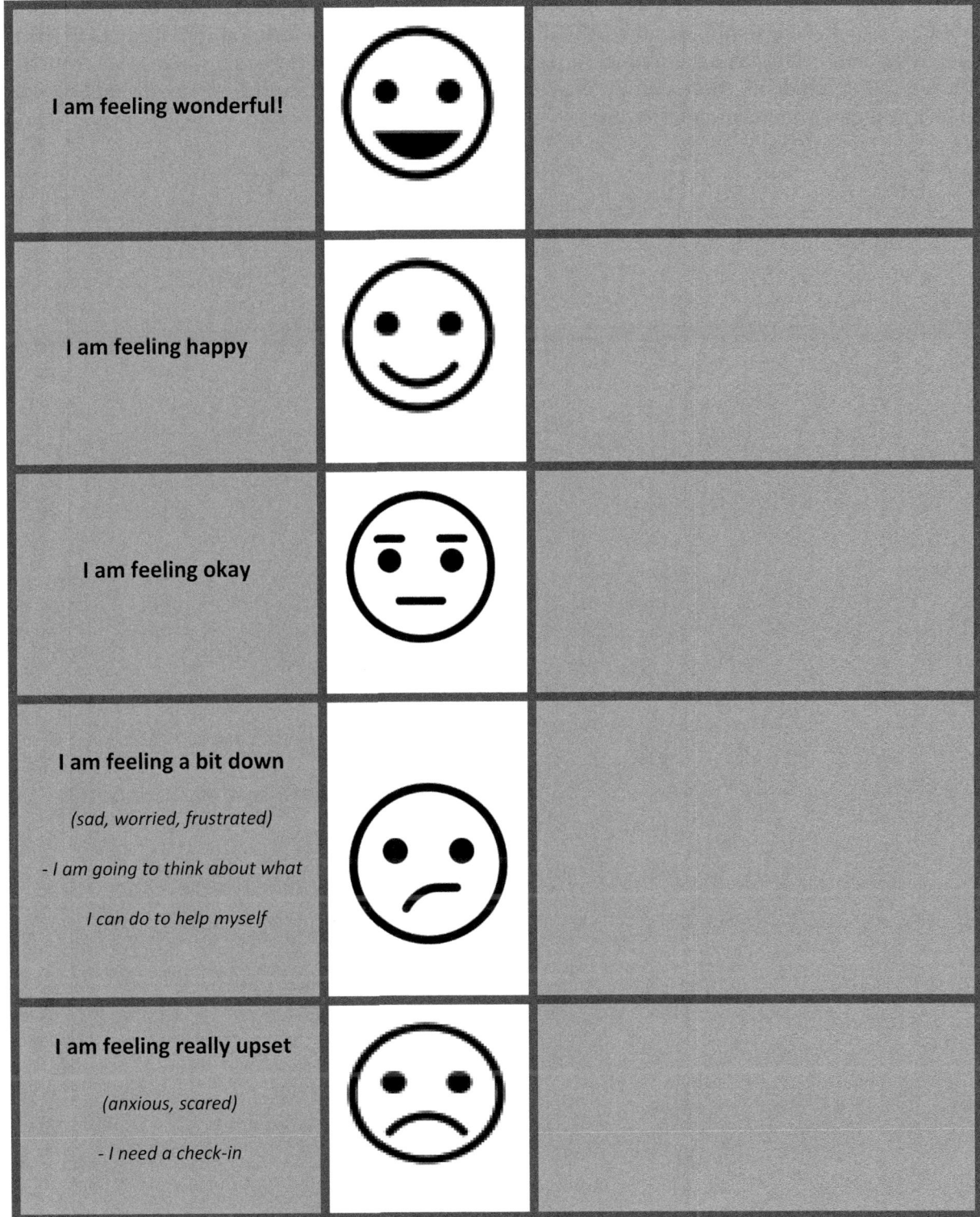

Figure 14.1 Emotion Check-In

understanding. Teachers become aware of how their students are doing and if they may need additional support and compassion that day. Also, by seeing classmates' emotion ratings, it can help them to feel more comfortable sharing their own feelings. The ratings also help to normalize all feelings, while reminding students those emotions are fluid and changeable, and how we are feeling can change minute to minute and day to day.

Calm Space

What It Is

A calm space is a spot in the classroom (or right outside of the room) where anyone can go when they are feeling overwhelmed by emotions and need a chance to re-set. The calming space offers a change in scenery, cues to support in reflecting upon emotions, and access to additional calming strategies. The calm space can be tailored to support the needs of the classroom. A calm space allows students who are struggling an opportunity to re-set and try calming down in a separate space. Sometimes walking away from the stress and worry can be helpful in re-grounding. In addition, a calm space may help to provide another layer of support for students and keep them close to the classroom and the instruction rather than them being at their desk and unfocused or leaving the room to get help elsewhere.

How It Looks

To set up the calm space, the following may be helpful suggestions:

- A space that provides low distraction but is still visible by the teacher. Consider the needs of your students and if it would be best for them to be in the class so they can still try to attend while at this space, or if it feels they need another option to leave the room and re-set. If both options can be helpful, two spaces could be considered.
- Available within the calm space:
  - Paper for drawing or writing.
  - Coloring pages and crayons, markers, or colored pencils.
  - Sensory/calming items such as: oil and water toy, squishy fidget, puzzle, headphones, and/or magnets.
  - A guiding plan for them such as in *Figure 14.2*.

For a successful introduction to a calm space, it's important that the students are taught the following:

- How to use the space – each student should be introduced to the space and then given an opportunity to try it out independently.
  - Explain, *"This space should be utilized when your body is feeling out of control."* Then ask, *"What indications might your body and mind give you that you need to use the calm space?"*
- Guidelines – rules should be outlined about how and when the space should be used.
  - When to use the space: the class should work together to identify when someone may need to utilize the calm space versus re-setting at their desk. Explain, *"You should use your body and mind to help you decide if you need a re-set at a new spot to feel calmer. Some clues you may get from your body are when you are moving a lot, or your heart is racing and it's hard to slow down. Your mind may have a hard time focusing."*
  - How to use the space: the following are some suggestions to consider as a class:
    - How many people can use this spot at once?
    - Is there a time limit? If so, how long?
    - How to use the items that are provided in the space?
  - Review the Calm Space Check In in *Figure 14.2*.
    - *"Notice how you are feeling when you first arrive at the calm space."*
    - *"Then, select a calming choice – writing or coloring, a fidget, reading, or a movement option"* (e.g., wall push-ups, seated push-ups, or moving a weighted ball back and forth).

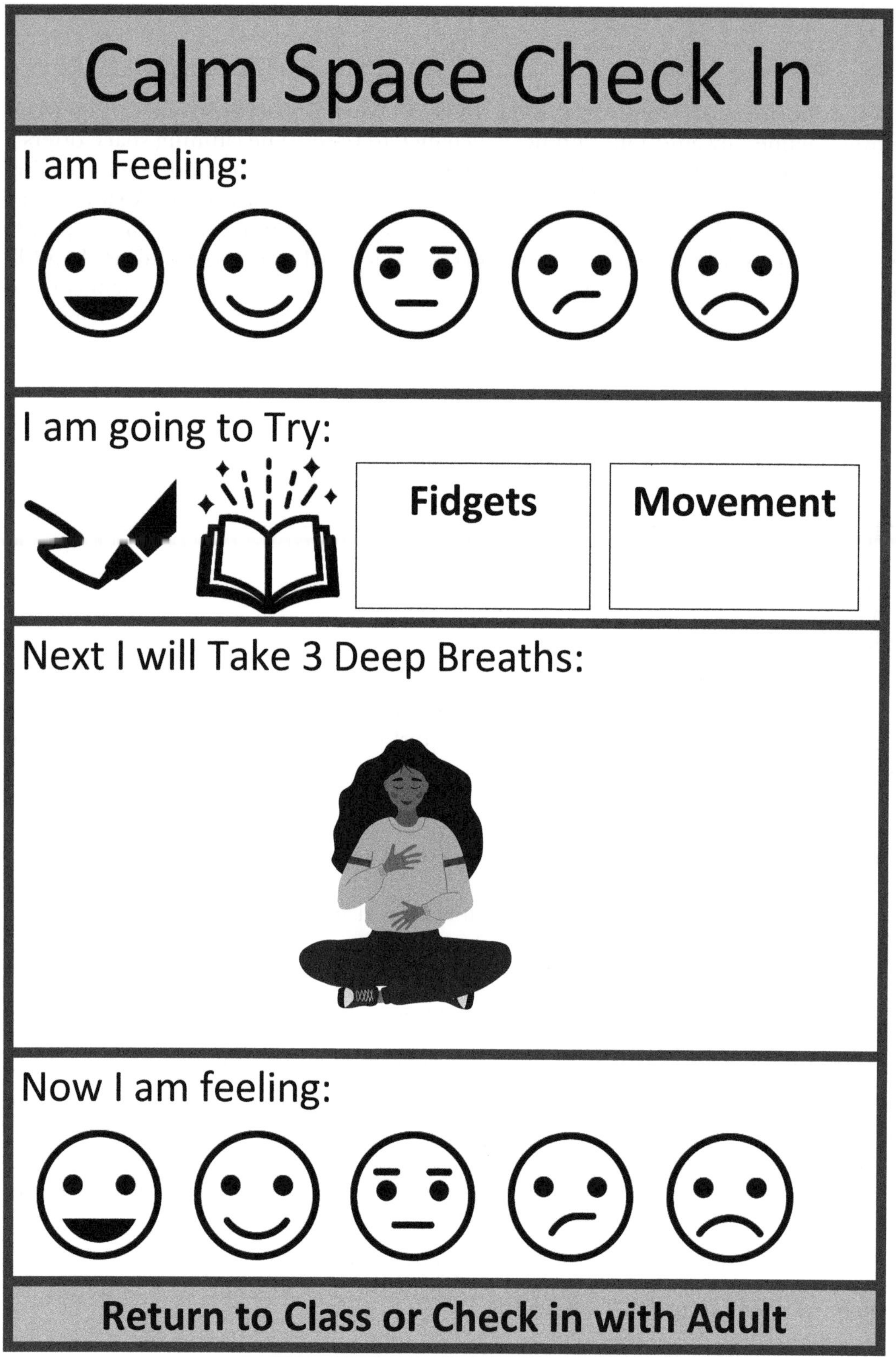

Calm Space Check In

I am Feeling:

I am going to Try:

Fidgets	Movement

Next I will Take 3 Deep Breaths:

Now I am feeling:

Return to Class or Check in with Adult

Figure 14.2 Calm Space Check-In

- ■ *"Next, take a deep breath using 4-7-8 breathing (breathe in for a count of four, hold your breath for seven seconds, and then breathe out while counting to eight) and repeat two more times."*
- ■ *"Finally, check back in regarding how you are feeling now. You should be feeling better, and if so, return to your seat. If you are not feeling better, come and talk with an adult for more strategies."*
- Practice – after introducing the space, take turns practicing utilizing this space. Tell students, *"We will be practicing using our Calm Space so that we feel more comfortable going there when our body and/ or mind need a re-set. I will tell you when it's your turn to try out the space. Let me know if any questions come up during your time and we can talk about them together."* Adults in the room can set a helpful example by showing how they are going to use the space and being very descriptive when they use it. For example, *"I am going to take a few minutes in our Calm Space because something just happened that has me feeling frustrated. I feel like I need a moment to re-set. You all can read for a few minutes."* This helps the students to see that even adults get upset and need to re-set at times.

Notes of Caution

- Do not: require students to use the space. You can gently suggest but should not force anyone to ever go to the space.
- Do not: use the calm space as a time out or as a way to punish a student. This will defeat the purpose of them utilizing this independently to help themselves calm down. If it is used as a consequence for their behavior, other students will also see this as an unfavorable space to go.
- Notice how often students are using the space and if anyone seems to be using it as an avoidance strategy. If this is happening, work with the student to understand what they might be trying to avoid and talk with them and any other necessary staff to create a plan that can help them to feel more successful in class and need the calm space less.

Daily Mindfulness

What It Is

Daily practices to cultivate mindfulness can support an entire class with gaining awareness of their emotions as well as promote feelings of calmness. Mindfulness-based practices can be used on a regular basis, or as needed when the classroom is high in energy and needs help to re-center. Most children and adolescents have shown an improvement in mental, behavioral, and physical outcomes when mindfulness-based interventions have been utilized (Ortiz & Sibinga, 2017). However, prior to utilizing these practices, students should be invited to participate in the practice but not forced.

If utilizing mindfulness-based practices on a regular basis within the classroom, the regular practice time could be determined based off of when the class may especially benefit from a break and re-focus opportunity. For instance, some classes struggle to continue with impulsive and loud behaviors when coming back in the room from recess. Therefore, after recess would be a good time to schedule a mindfulness-based practice. Another time is often right away in the morning if students are coming to school feeling stressed and worried about the day. Really any time of day can be an opportunity to practice mindfulness. The following are strategies that can be used to support the whole class:

- Class set up:
  - Playing calm music during work.
  - Dimming lights and including more lamps and string lights throughout the room.
  - Calm colors and thoughtful room decoration.
    - A room with calm features that mimic the warmth of home can feel relaxing.
    - A room with a lot of bright colors and lots to look at can make it difficult to focus and feel overwhelming.
  - Using a chime to gain student attention.

Classroom Intention

What It Is

The Classroom Intention Script provides a reminder to students that they are cared for in the classroom. This practice helps to promote positivity, connection, and reflection. This may be especially helpful to utilize at the beginning of the day. If utilizing with specific students, it can be a helpful script for those who may feel especially nervous about being at school, and/or are struggling to focus in the moment due to worries from home.

How It Looks

Read this script (*Box 14.1*) aloud to students in a calm, slow voice. Pause throughout so that the practice is not rushed and students are allowed time to sit with their thoughts. Also note that for this intention script, you can alter the wording of safe, loved, and appreciated to something else that may align more closely with words you use to help students feel cared for.

Box 14.1

Classroom Intention

Classroom Intention Script

"I invite you to find a comfortable seated position. Take a deep breath in through your nose, as you breathe out through your mouth, close your eyes or gaze downward at the floor. Breathe in deeply through your nose again … hold your breath … and now breathe slowly out from your mouth. Right now in this moment, you are safe … you are loved … and you are appreciated. Repeat in your mind … I am safe … I am loved … and I am appreciated … Again, I am safe … I am loved … and I am appreciated … Things may arise today that challenge your thinking and make you feel worried, scared, frustrated, or upset. At that moment remind yourself that you always have your breath. Breathe in … hold … breathe out. Breathe in … hold … breathe out. Repeat to yourself one last time, I am safe, I am loved, and I am appreciated. Breathe in … breathe out and begin to bring your awareness back to the room. When you are ready, slowly open your eyes."

Discussion questions:

- How did that feel?
- What did you notice during that practice that you didn't previously notice?
- When might be good times for you to remind yourself of these intentions?
- Do you have other intentions that can be helpful to remind yourself?

Breath Awareness

What It Is

The Breath Awareness Script (*Box 14.2*) provides a mindful breathing activity to promote awareness of what is happening within us as well as around us. Oftentimes, our mind is thinking about many different things – maybe something that already happened, or something that's going to happen, or our mind is making connections based on what we're hearing around us. This activity helps in re-centering the mind and bringing focus back to the present. It helps to serve as a reminder that although our days may be chaotic and we may come into contact with obstacles, we always have the constant of our breath.

How It Looks

Throughout this practice, be sure to pause frequently and talk slowly as a way to allow the student(s) the opportunity for their mind to wander, and then bring it back through grounding themselves with their breath and your words. The practice could be shorter or longer based on the age and capacity for mindfulness of your students. The awareness activity can be done by adding more pauses and longer or shorter breaks.

Box 14.2

Breath Awareness

Breath Awareness Script

"Find a comfortable seated or lying down position. Close your eyes or gaze downward. Now breathe in and feel your breath fill your stomach and notice its expansion. Hold your breath in your stomach… and now breathe out and notice the air traveling up and out of your mouth. Breathe in … hold … and breathe out. For the next five minutes, you are going to focus on your breathing. Right now, in this moment, you have nothing that needs to be done or accomplished. Right now, you are able to focus on the now. You may breathe normally. As you notice a thought arise acknowledge that thought like you would a cloud floating past, with awareness but without a response, reaction, or judgment. Then bring your attention back to your breath. Breathing in … and out. Many times, when a thought arises, we can get lost in the thought – considering what next action should happen. To be mindful involves observing the thoughts that arise with awareness and acceptance but not action or judgment. Breathe in … breathe out … (pause and allow the students to continue their practice independently for about a minute) *… If you notice your mind wandering again, find grounding in my voice and your breath. Breathe in … hold … breathe out. Notice how*

the breath feels throughout your body – how does it impact your heart, your legs, your arms, your mind? Breathe in ... breathe out (pause for another minute). As you hear sounds in the distance, it's ok to become aware and observe them, and then bring your attention back to your breath. Breathe in ... hold ... breathe out... Now begin to bring your awareness back to the room. On your next breath, slowly open your eyes."

Discussion questions:

- How did it feel to pay attention to your breath in that way?
- What did you notice during that practice that you weren't previously aware of?
- Do you find it easy or challenging to not react or respond to thoughts that occur? Please explain.
- How might this type of practice be helpful in everyday life?

Positive Moment Visualization

What It Is

The Positive Moment Visualization (*Box 14.3*) can be used at any time of day and with any group of students. The objective for this visualization is to support the student(s) in focusing on a memory that can bring them happiness. The intent is to teach students the practice of savoring positive moments.

How It Looks

When reading this visualization and following up with the discussion questions, remind students that they do not need to share, and this can be a private memory for them. You may also support them with their memory by prefacing this moment by saying, *"I'm going to ask you to think about a positive moment in your life, this means that I want you to think about a time that made you feel happy. This time might be something really big like going to Disney World. Or, it may be something that can happen any day of the week like going for a walk outside with your family."* Be sure to pause throughout reading so that the student has space with their own thoughts where you aren't always speaking. This allows them to potentially notice things that you aren't directing them to notice.

Box 14.3

Positive Moment Visualization

Positive Moment Script

"Find a comfortable seated position. Breathe in ... and out ... Gently close your eyes or gaze downward. Breathe in ... hold ... Breathe out. Breathe in ... and breathe out. Now, take a moment to think about a moment where you felt happy ... Your thought may be of a special moment, or an everyday occurrence that makes you feel happy to remember and think about ... Consider this moment ... notice where you are ... what do you see? ... What do you hear? ... Who is with you? ... Are there any certain smells you notice? ... Pay attention to how your body feels ... What thoughts are coming into your mind? ... How do you feel? ... In this moment you are happy ... you are safe ... Breathe in ... Breathe out ... Savor this moment and remember that when times are challenging, you can go to this space and this memory ... and feel happy and safe ... When you are ready, bring your awareness back to the room ... Take another deep breath in ... hold ... and breathe out ... now open your eyes."

Discussion questions:

- Would anyone like to share about what came to mind for them?
- What was it about this experience that stood out to you in your mind as a positive moment?
- How did it feel to think back on a memory in this way?
- Do you think you would be able to think of a positive memory in this way again if you were feeling down? How might this type of visualization be helpful?

Mindful Walking

What It Is

Mindful Walking (*Box 14.4*) is a practice that incorporates movement into mindfulness. Walking in a mindful way promotes awareness of surroundings as well as specific attention toward the physical act of walking. Oftentimes, when walking, we are walking with a purpose and do not pay much attention to what it feels like for our feet to hit the ground, or our body to propel forward. This practice supports engagement for those who may struggle to sit still for a reflective mindfulness practice.

How It Looks

The Mindful Walking script (*Box 14.4*) should be read prior to the student(s) beginning the mindful walking practice. Students should listen to this reading in its entirety before getting started. The practice can be done inside or outside but should not be confined to a small space like a classroom. You may decide to also add parameters on where is ok to walk and where is too far so that you are able to keep track of the student(s). A time limit should be given so students know when they should return.

Box 14.4

Mindful Walking

Mindful Walking Script

"Today we are going to practice being mindful while walking. This type of exercise includes paying attention to your movement in a mindful way while also observing your surroundings. We are all going to walk for the next ten minutes in a mindful way. (Next, state where this will be happening and any parameters). Your challenge is to walk more slowly and with awareness. This can be done by paying attention to your breathing ... how does your breathing change as you move? Be aware of your environment ... recognize what is around you as you walk. Notice the colors ... the plants ... the smell. Observe how your body feels to move as you walk. What does it feel like for your feet to hit the ground? ... Notice how your arms swing as your legs move... While you are walking if you notice your mind wandering, observe that thought and then return to the moment and your awareness of what is around you."

Discussion questions:

- How did it feel to walk in this way?
- What did you become aware of while walking mindfully that you are not typically aware of when you walk?
- What did you find most challenging about this exercise?

Loving-Kindness Meditation

What It Is

Loving-Kindness Meditation is focused on sending and receiving love and kindness. This practice involves visualization to support sending and receiving positivity and compassion. Practicing kindness toward others can support feeling more connected and less lonely (Hutcherson, Seppala, & Gross, 2008).

How It Looks

The Loving-Kindness Meditation (*Box 14.5*) can be utilized as a way to help promote positive feelings and connection. In the classroom, this practice could be used at any time, but especially when students may be feeling down or when the class is in conflict. The Loving-Kindness Meditation helps to remind us that we each are similar in some way and we all want to feel love and kindness. Before beginning the meditation, have all students get into a large circle, preferably seated but standing can work as well.

Box 14.5

Loving-Kindness Meditation

Loving-Kindness Meditation Script

"Everyone take a deep breath in … and out … Now close your eyes or gaze downward at the floor. Think about someone that you love very much … Picture this person in your mind and what you love about them … Now, we are going to send them positive wishes.

- *Quietly whisper:*
    - *I wish you happiness.*
    - *I wish you kindness.*
    - *I wish you to be free from pain.*

Next, think about the person to your left. Picture this person in your mind. Consider that they have things that make them happy as well as things that make them feel sad. They have good days as well as bad days. As you think about this person, send them your compassion.

- *Quietly whisper aloud:*
    - *I wish you happiness.*
    - *I wish you kindness.*
    - *I wish you to be free from pain.*

Now, take a deep breath in … and out … Consider the person to your right. Form a picture of this person in your mind. Remember, that just like you, they feel happy some times and sad at other times. Their life too is full of ups and downs. As you consider this person, send them well wishes.

- *Quietly whisper:*
    - *I wish you happiness.*
    - *I wish you kindness.*
    - *I wish you to be free from pain.*

Finally, take another deep breath in … and out … and picture yourself. Remember that you are human and can make amazing things happen, but also are allowed to make mistakes. As you think of yourself, consider what you love about yourself … What makes you unique? … Now, send yourself some self-love.

- *Quietly whisper:*
    - *I wish myself happiness.*
    - *I wish myself kindness.*
    - *I wish myself to be free from pain.*

Take another deep breath in … hold … and breathe out. Begin to bring your attention back to the room and your surroundings. On your next in breath, open your eyes."

Discussion questions:

- How did it feel to participate in this activity?
- What thoughts did you have as your peer was wishing you well?
- What did you find most difficult about this practice?

Short Mindful Moments

What It Is

In addition to intentional mindful meditation practices, Mindful Moments (*Table 14.1*) can be incorporated throughout the day in any activity. As a way to support student awareness within the moment and with their breath, the following short Mindful Moments in *Table 14.1* can be helpful to utilize in the classroom.

Table 14.1 Mindful Moments

Practice	How it Looks
Purposeful standing and sitting	While raising to a standing position, do so very slowly and pay attention to the sensations in your body. Take a deep breath in and out at the top and then very slowly sit back down. While working toward sitting, observe how your muscles feel – are they similar or different to when you were standing?
Singing bowl/ chime	Utilize a singing bowl or chime to make a high-pitched noise for students to hear. Ask them to raise their hand when they no longer hear the noise. This allows for them to mindfully focus on the noise and also helps to make them aware of how we may hear the sound stop at different points in time (some students may be able to hear the pitch longer while others cannot).
Calm listening	Turn on calm music without words in the background while students are working independently. This can support students in feeling calm and focused as it can drown out other noises in the classroom.
Body check-in	Multiple times throughout the day, ask students to stop and recognize how they are feeling. Remind them that all feelings are ok, and feelings tend to change over time. As they check in on how they are feeling, share some options that can be used to support them in feeling calm, such as deep breathing or some body movement.
Intention setting	At the start of the day or class period, take a moment where everyone is calm and quiet. Ask students to think about what their goal is for the class and how they will attain that goal. Take another minute of quiet breathing and then start the class. At the end of the class, take a minute for students to quietly reflect on how they did working toward the goal they had set for themselves.
Breathing ball	Use an Expandable Breathing Ball to support a visualization of breathing deeply in and out. Slowly, pull the ball outward to a count of four to create a large ball shape while everyone breathes in. Hold the ball in that shape for a count of seven and then, slowly push the ball back together for a count of eight. Repeat this activity until the class appears more calm.

Deep Breathing Graphics

Deep breathing is something that can be done to support the body in feeling calm. Deep breathing is a way that we can purposely work to regulate intense feelings. There are many different kinds of breathing exercises and practices. At the core of each practice is the same idea, which includes slowing down the breath while being intentional about breathing. Below are some options that could be used within the classroom. The figures are meant to be utilized as posters to remind about deep breathing options for reference in the classroom.

Square Breathing

What It Is

Square breathing (*Figure 14.3*) uses the shape (a square) to help support slowing down and guiding the breath. Breathing while tracing a shape can help to focus the mind through multiple ways (physical movement and thought). In addition, breathing with the support of a picture can help to slow down the breath and then allow to support a calmer feeling across the body and the mind.

How It Looks

With square breathing, you can use an actual square (or rectangle) to guide your practice, or you can create your own with your finger in the air or on a surface. If using an actual square (or rectangle) figure such as a door, a tile, or a wall poster, students can be taught to look at that figure but still keep their distance and follow their breathing using that item as a guide. Students can also be taught to go up to that item and trace it right there (this option may be more appropriate for younger students). In addition to having an actual square (or rectangle) in the room to support visualization, students may also prefer to just draw their own while following square breathing and have their finger in the air or on a surface. Different options should be practiced with the class when introducing square breathing.

Breathe In Positivity and Breathe Out Negativity

What It Is

Another way to promote focusing of breath and mind is through a visualization where you breathe in positivity and breathe out negativity. The focus of breathing in this way is to work on being aware of what is allowed into the mind and then releasing those that are hurtful to overall well-being.

How It Looks

In this practice, students should begin by considering how they might fill their body with positivity and then visualize that happening with each in breath. On the exhale, students are asked to breathe out any negativity or bad things that they are holding within themselves. Figure 14.4 provides a visualization for this practice.

Square Breathing

- Breathe in as you trace the left side of the square from bottom to top.

- Hold your breath as you trace the top of the square.

- Breathe out as you trace the right side of the square.

- Then, hold as you trace the bottom and last part of the square.

- Repeat.

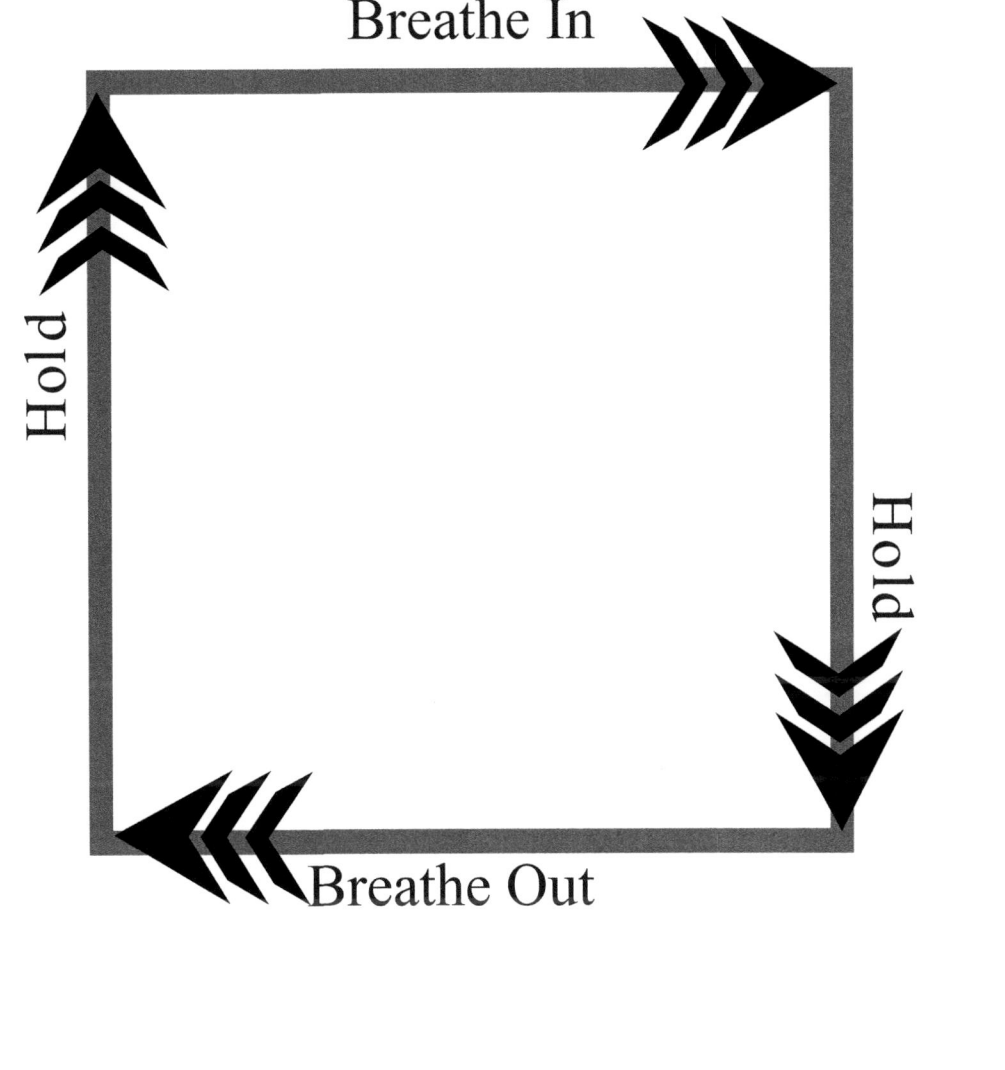

Figure 14.3 Square Breathing

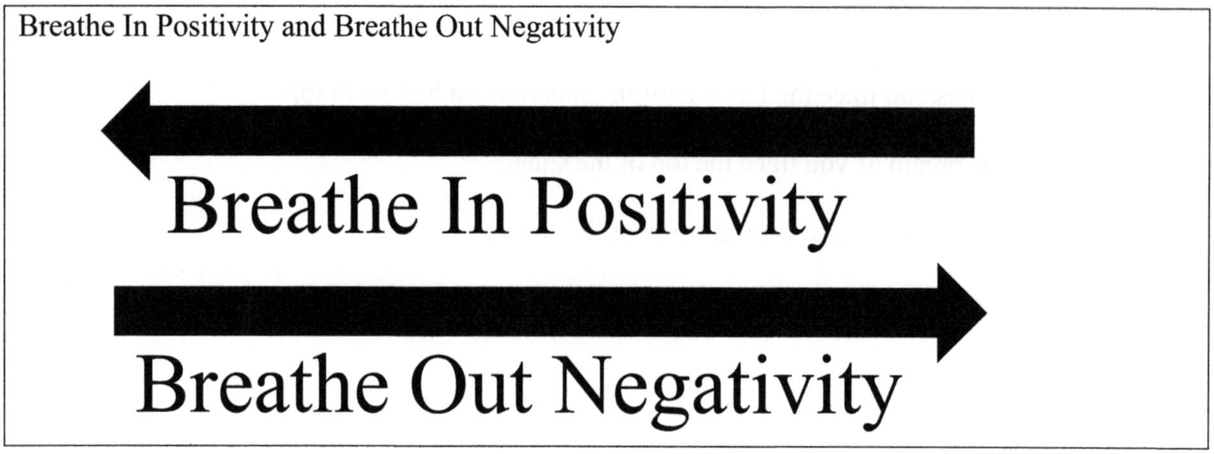

Figure 14.4 Breathe In Positivity and Breathe Out Negativity

Accommodations

Anxiety can impact student learning as well as performance. Therefore, it is important that students with anxiety have access to appropriate accommodations to support their capacity to learn and connect with others throughout the school day. Some possible accommodations for a team to consider for students with anxiety have been outlined below.

- Preferential seating – e.g., seated away from distractions, close to supportive peer.
- Breaks (e.g., mindful calm time by self, walking hallway) – when feeling overwhelmed and/or scheduled throughout the day – work with the student to come up with a signal for when breaks are needed so that they don't need to verbally request a break.
- Additional time on tests and assignments (e.g., expected to complete work by end of quarter; additional time on standardized tests).
- Testing in a quiet/separate environment.
- Provide advance notice when changes to the daily schedule occur.
- Break down assignments and tasks into smaller chunks.
- Check in with the student privately for understanding of learning.
- Allow use of notes for tests and quizzes (e.g., the student is allowed the use of one page, front and back, to support them during a test or quiz).
- Use of audiobooks.
- Pre-created plan to support student when returning from an absence (e.g., homework is forgiven, homework is reduced, or student is allowed time to stay at school to complete missed work).
- Reduction in amount of work expected (homework and assessments) – may consider a time limit in which the student doesn't work on homework longer than a certain period of time.
- Determine communication system to discreetly communicate when the child is feeling anxious and needs a break or to talk with designated adult.
- Identify a point person at school for the student to meet with if feeling anxious.
- Foreshadow any changes to the schedule while being as specific as possible about expectations surrounding the change (e.g., we will be seeing a movie after lunch tomorrow so we will not have our afternoon classes. We will be walking to the theater and will not be eating any snacks while we are there).
- Provide reminders when it is getting close to a transition time and what can be done if not finished (e.g., you have five minutes left to finish up working on the math problem, if it's not complete, you can work on it during study hall).
- Social anxiety:
  - Opportunity to give class speech one-on-one with teacher or make a video tape to share with the class or teacher.
  - Do not call on the student unless they raise their hand.
  - Opportunity to leave class early between transitions to avoid busy hallways.

- Specific phobia:
  - Modify schedules and environments to support increased comfort (e.g., if the student is fearful of germs, consider an individual stall bathroom for use by the student).

- Panic disorder/student has panic attacks:
  - Share signs of panic attack happening with staff along with individualized plan of how to support the student if they are experiencing a panic attack (e.g., the student should report to the office and the office will call a designated person close to the student to support them with coping with their intense feelings of panic).

- Post-traumatic stress disorder:
  - ○ If triggers for the student are known, they should be outlined in the student plan with ideas for how to offset the trauma-inducing trigger. (e.g.; noise reducing headphones/earplugs, placement considerations, tone of voice).

These accommodations are general examples that may be useful for students who have anxiety. Any plan to support a student should be created with the student's needs in mind and based on their individual circumstances. Parents, teachers, and the student are often the best at identifying what could be most useful to support access to learning.

Individualized Education Plan (IEP) Goals

Students with anxiety who also have support through an IEP may benefit from goals focused on supporting their growth and progress with worry and coping strategies. Goals that may be especially appropriate could include working toward emotional awareness, emotion regulation, and coping mechanisms.

- Emotional awareness:
    - In moments of high anxiety, _____ will use pre-taught physical and thought clues to identify how they are feeling and share this feeling with a trusted adult _____% of observed occurrences.
    - _____ will accurately identify their feelings using a feelings check-in _____% of times with accuracy matched by a trusted school staff member rating.

- Emotion regulation:
    - _____ will show self-awareness when needing additional support in working through a problem by requesting to talk to a trusted adult independently without prompts in ____% of occurrences.
    - In times of heightened emotions, _____ will identify a pre-taught coping strategy to use, and after finished with the strategy, will return to the class with a calm demeanor in _____% of occurrences.

- Coping mechanisms:
    - When _____ is experiencing emotion dysregulation, they will independently choose a pre-taught coping strategy to support in feeling calm _____% of observed occurrences.
    - During times of stress where the focus is on the negative, _____ will challenge their thoughts and consider what is most likely to happen versus what is the worst thing that will happen. Progress will be measured weekly and is expected to show a reduction in initial self-report ratings from _____ to _____ (ratings of 1–10 with 10 expressing expertise in challenging thoughts).
    - _____ will be able to verbally identify ____ strategies by the end of the school year that they can use when feeling anxious.
    - As a way to improve feelings of anxiety, _____ will utilize stress reduction practices ____ times per week and keep track of them in a journal from which they share weekly with a staff member.

Works Cited

Hutcherson, C. A., Seppala, E. M., & Gross, J. J. (2008). Loving-kindness meditation increases social connectedness. *Emotion, 8*(5), 720–724.

Ortiz, R., & Sibinga, E. M. (2017). The role of mindfulness in reducing the adverse effects of childhood stress and trauma. *Children, 4*(3), 16.

15 Continued Support for Home

The following are additional support options that can be shared with parents based on their individual child's needs and favorite coping strategies. Above all else, parents can be reminded of the importance of reinforcing to their child that all emotions are acceptable. Oftentimes, people with anxiety are told that when they have a negative thought, they should just think of something else or somehow try to get rid of that thought. The focus in this book is to become aware and accepting of the thoughts that occur, and when we notice that we are focusing on more negative thinking or worry that is unlikely to happen, we challenge the thought. Student's guardians are invited to support their children in this process. The following family practices are described in this chapter:

- Gratitude Reflection.
- Calm Space.
- Family Mindfulness.
- A Worry Box.
- What Went Well Today.
- Specific Praise Each Night.
- What Is Something You're Looking Forward to Today?

DOI: 10.4324/9781003324782-15

Gratitude Reflection

What It Is

A gratitude reflection offers the opportunity to think back on the positive aspects of the day.

How It Looks

Use this reflection guide (*Table 15.1*) to share about moments of gratitude from each day. Set aside time each day to reflect on moments of gratitude with your child. *Figure 15.1* can be used for your child to write down their reflections, or as a guide for a reminder of what questions to ask verbally. While taking time to do this with your child, you can participate as well in answering the questions. This activity can be a one-on-one reflection, an individual reflection, or a family reflection.

Gratitude Reflection

Monday
I am grateful for this person:

Friday
I am grateful for this person:

I am thankful that this happened today:

I am thankful that this happened today:

Tuesday
I am grateful for this person:

Saturday
I am grateful for this person:

I am thankful that this happened today:

I am thankful that this happened today:

Wednesday
I am grateful for this person:

Sunday
I am grateful for this person:

I am thankful that this happened today:

I am thankful that this happened today:

Thursday
I am grateful for this person:

I am thankful that this happened today:

Table 15.1 Gratitude Reflection

Calm Space Check In

I am Feeling:

I am going to Try:

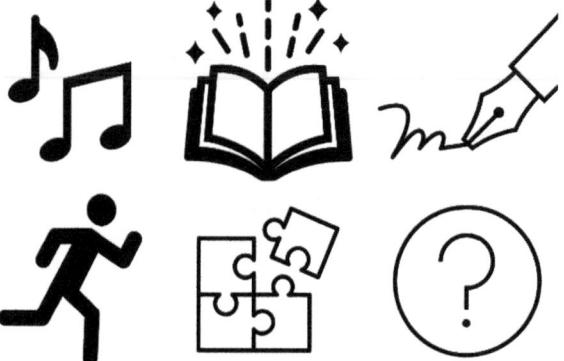

Next I will Take 3 Deep Breaths:

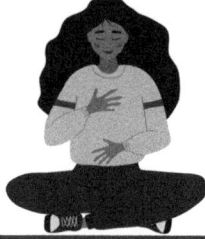

Now I am feeling:

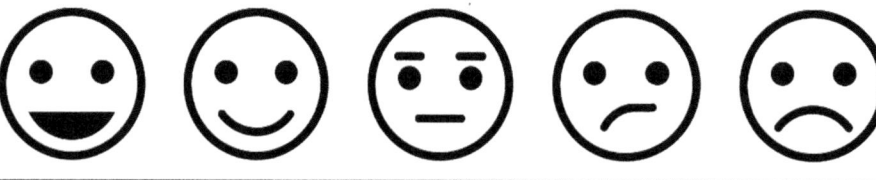

Leave Calming Space or Check-in with Trusted Adult

Figure 15.1 Calm Space Check In

Calm Space

What It Is

A calm space is a space that can be used for your child to re-set themselves when they are feeling anxious. This space offers a chance for children and adolescents to be by themselves and with things that can help them to regulate their emotions. A calm space is intended NOT as a punishment, but instead as a place where your child is allowed to feel what they are feeling without judgment. A calm space also offers children and adolescents to take the time they need to get themselves feeling calmer and more stable. The calming corner offers a change in scenery, cues to support in reflecting upon emotions, and access to additional calming strategies.

How It Looks

The calm space can be tailored to support the needs of your child. To set up the calming space, the following may be helpful suggestions:

- A space that provides low distraction. If possible, it's ideal that it is not a multi-use space that may be entered upon by others in the family. A space that may work best would be a closet, a corner in the child's bedroom, or a space in an office or spare bedroom that is rarely used.
- Something that makes the space distinct and separate from the larger space such as a chair, a room divider, a curtain, a blanket covering the space, or a sign.
- Available within the calm space:
  - Paper for drawing or writing.
  - Coloring pages and crayons, markers, or colored pencils.
  - Sensory/calming items chosen by the child. You might offer the following as suggestions: fidgets, puzzles, books, music, pictures, or a favorite item that supports them in feeling calm. Avoid technology if possible unless a calm relaxation app or tool is being utilized.
  - A guiding plan for them such as in *Figure 15.1*.

For the calm space to be utilized when needed and as expected by your child, the following are important points to keep in mind:

- Show the child that you respect their time in their calm space, e.g., *"I see that you're in your calm space, would you like me to shut the door so that we aren't too loud out here?"* OR *"How are the items that you have in your calm space working for you? Is there anything else that you think might work well?"*
- Don't pressure your child to explain why they've chosen to use the calm space or what they did while they were in the calm space.
- Guidelines – it would be especially helpful if you outlined any rules that may be applicable to this space and potentially have your child's input into what guidelines would be appropriate. Some considerations may be:
  - When to use the space? – Are there certain times when it is not ok for them to utilize this space, and they can instead do something else to calm their body like deep breathing? (e.g., when it's time to leave the house, at bedtime).
  - How to use the space:
    - Is there a time limit for use of the space?
    - If you are needed for something in the house, what is the expectation for leaving the calming space. For example: leave 1 minute after parents call that it is supper time.
    - Is there anything that is not allowed in the space?
    - Will rewards be used for use of the space? – kids could earn points toward something each time they use the space if this would support its usage.

- o Review the Calm Space Check In (*Figure 15.1*) and ask if this might be useful for your child. If they would prefer, they can create their own instead. You can explain the check in with them.

  - *"Notice how you are feeling when you first arrive at the calm space."*
  - *"Then, select a calming choice – listening to music, reading, journaling, movement, a puzzle, or something else that you find calming."*
  - *"Next, take a deep breath using 4-7-8 breathing (breathe in for a count of four, hold your breath for seven seconds, and then breathe out while counting to eight) and repeat two more times."*
  - *"Finally, check back in regarding how you are feeling now. You should be feeling better, and if so, that can be your indication that you're ready to leave. If you are not feeling better, come and find me or someone else that you think might be able to help."*

Notes of Caution

- Do not: require your child to use the space if they do not want to. You can gently suggest but should not force anyone to ever go to the space.
- Do not: use the calm space as a time out or as a way to punish your child. This will defeat the purpose of them utilizing this independently to help themselves calm down.
- Notice how your child uses the space and if it ever seems to be used as an avoidance strategy. If this is happening, work with your child to understand what they might be trying to avoid and talk with them to try and create a plan from which both of you agree.

Family Mindfulness

What It Is

Practicing mindfulness can help your child to focus on the moment without reacting to thoughts or making judgment of themselves in some way. Mindfulness is a way of helping to practice sitting with thoughts and allowing them to pass without always feeling a need to change them, act on them, or judge them (Bishop et al., 2004). Learning to use the mind in this way can help your child to feel more at ease when anxious feelings and situations arise. Utilizing mindfulness as a family can support your child in seeing emotional and mental health as being just as important as our physical health. Just like our children understand us as prioritizing our strength and physical well-being when we are exercising, this helps them to see us prioritizing our mental well-being.

How It Looks

Mindfulness is something that could be scheduled on a regular basis within your family, or it is something that you can simply incorporate into your daily activities. If scheduling mindfulness, consider if your family would like to independently practice mindfulness or practice together.

- Scheduled practice:
  - Independent or as a family:
    - Independent practice: if your child prefers independent practice, you can still schedule a family time for mindful meditation but each one of you could work on your mindfulness independently in your own space.
    - Family practice: if the preference is a mindfulness practice as a family, you could all share a space and utilize the same form of mindful meditation.
  - How to plan this practice:
    - Time: consider what time of the day can work best for everyone and is likely to be low distraction each day.
    - Where: a quiet space should be used that is limited with distractions. You may choose to have a rug or something comfortable to sit on or lie down on. In addition, your space may include a few objects that are important to you and can support you with your focus of being in the moment. This space shall not only serve as comfort but also a cue to your brain to start your practice.
    - Days: what days of the week would work best to practice. You might try every day if possible, but if that feels too daunting, consider three days a week. Determine what days will offer the best opportunity to ensure your practice is able to occur.
    - Prior to beginning your practice, it can be helpful to set an intention for your time together. For example, you may come together and say a word that is your focus throughout your mindful practice (e.g., breath – I will remain focused on my breath and when I notice I'm not I will gently bring my mind back to my breath).
    - What will you use to support your mindfulness practice? Below are some options that you can consider, remember that the way you choose to practice mindfulness can be personal and unique to you.
      - Mindful meditation apps to utilize on a digital device.
      - Listening to calming music and working to focus on the moment by coloring or drawing. Whenever your mind wanders, bring it back to your breath and the act of drawing/coloring.
      - Yoga/movement as a way to coordinate the breath with the mind and body.

- After practicing mindfulness, you may offer an opportunity to share how you now feel and what you liked or found challenging about the practice (e.g., I found it very calming to focus on my breathing, but I noticed I had lots of thoughts about something that is going to happen later today keep popping up for me – that was a challenge as I was distracted a lot).

- Incorporated into family activities:

  o Consider bringing up awareness of what you see, hear, feel, smell, and can touch while doing activities together as a family. The following activities are examples of what could be used but not all inclusive as there are endless ways to incorporate mindfulness.

  o Walking outside – create a journal log or verbally share what sounds are noticed, what new creatures are found, and all the different shades of green, brown, and blue that are seen.

  o Play a game together – share out loud what feelings you're aware of while playing a game. Express what you notice within and outside of your body.

    - For example:

      □ Hide and seek – I notice my heart is racing when I am hiding and trying not to be found. I could hear the seeker's footsteps when they were trying to find me. What did you notice?

      □ Chess – each piece is very smooth. The colors appear to be all the same on each side but I'm noticing that the shades of the brown are a little different on each piece. I wonder what the factory looks like that made these pieces. What do you notice?

      □ A game of basketball – I notice the ridges on the basketball and that I like the lines to be a certain way when I go for a shot. What do you notice?

      □ Family car ride – play a game of I spy and see what you can notice in terms of certain colors and sounds.

      □ Put together a puzzle as a family – for those who struggle to move past tough thoughts, a distraction such as a puzzle can offer the perfect opportunity for a project to divert thinking away from worries and focus together on completing the puzzle.

A Worry Box

What It Is

A worry box is a box where your child can place their worries. They can write down a thought that is bothering them and then place it inside of the worry box. Once the thought is written down and placed inside of the box, the worry can be let go of, and thoughts can focus on something else.

How It Looks

While creating the worry box, consider the following suggestions for implementation:

- Encourage your child to decorate their worry box on their own. Encourage them to make it unique to them.
- Determine a good spot to place the worry box. Is it best in their room where only they have access to the box? Or would they prefer it be in a common area so that maybe others in the family can contribute?
- Explain that the worry box is where they can place their worries by writing about them or drawing them and then putting that piece of paper into the box. Share that the idea is that once they share their worry, they can move on to think about something different.
- Offer that the worries can be shredded, or a time can be made for you to read the worries with your child on a regular basis (no more frequently than once per day).
  - If reading the worries with your child, reinforce discussion. Talk about times when something felt like a big worry, but then over time now it seems to be smaller (e.g., on Monday, they were really worried about something embarrassing they said at lunch, but now as you discuss it on Wednesday, they realize no one really cared and it wasn't that big of a deal).
  - Check in to see how your child would most like you involved when reading through worries together and note that this may change based on each worry or by each day. Ask questions such as, *"Would you like me to read the worry, or would you like to read the worry?"* and *"Would you like my advice or for me to just listen?"*
  - Provide empathy always. Before jumping too quickly to an idea on solving their worry, make sure to empathize with how they felt by summarizing their feeling back to them. For example, *"Oh yes, I'm sure this really made you feel embarrassed. I wish you hadn't had to go through that experience."*

What Went Well Today

What It Is

Helping your child to focus on the positive can help to support their overall resiliency (Smith Harvey, 2007). For this reason, it is important to help to promote savoring positive moments in our children. This can be done by reminding them of pieces of their day that went well.

How It Looks

The following activities can be helpful in checking in about positive thinking throughout the day. Ask your child about a favorite moment from their day. Oftentimes, the question is asked, "How was your day?" and the answer includes, "Fine" or some other short and one-worded response. Instead, ask your child one of these more specific questions that may invoke a more thorough response.

- What was the best part of your day today?
- Tell me about the funniest thing that happened today?
- How did you show kindness to someone else today?
- What is something you did that you feel proud of today?
- What is something you're grateful for from today?
- Who are three people you smiled at today?
- What is something funny one of your teachers said today?
- What was the best part of your lunch today?

Specific Praise Each Night

What It Is

Annika Swenson, a mother of three and cancer researcher, created the idea of specific praise for children by using it each night with her own young children (personal communication, August 6, 2021). When using specific praise, your child is told what they did that was positive during the day. As a way to close each night, share three positive things about your child from that day. This is an opportunity for your child to challenge any negative thinking of themselves while hearing positives that someone they love notices about them. Sharing these three things at night before bed also helps for the evening to end in a positive way. Although this is a simple task, a few pointers may support positive acknowledgments in being something your child looks forward to each night.

How It Looks

- Determine where and when you will do this with your child. Plan for a routine that works well with what you already utilize for bedtime. Consider, is it done in their room before they fall asleep? Is it something done before they go into their room? Is it always the same adult, or are there times it is someone else?
- Praise their actions, not them as a person. For example: you're a hard worker versus you're so smart. This distinction feels small but is big, because being a hard worker suggests that this is an action that is more changeable and within their control. While smart can feel more set in stone and something that is less movable.
- Share specific and novel examples and characteristics whenever possible. For example, "You showed so much responsibility today by remembering everything you needed to take to school and reminding me not to forget your permission slip!"
- Focus all your attention on them when providing them with their three positives. If your phone rings, let it ring. If you get a text, leave it until later. Make sure this time is focused just on your child.
- For children that thrive with physical touch and closeness, squeeze a finger for each characteristic that is shared.
- Have your child repeat back what you said (at least the main phrase) (e.g., guardian says, "You were so kind today when you helped your brother with his homework," child would respond, "I was so kind."
- Have your child make up one of their own to say about themselves as a person after you've said three. If they share something like, "I'm nice," ask them for an example of how they were nice. Push a little bit so that they can share specifics and really work to begin believing and seeing these amazing things they are doing in daily life.

What Is Something You're Looking Forward to Today?

What It Is

A check in with your child to set up the day in a positive mindset. Asking about something your child is looking forward to can re-set the morning and help to send children and adolescents off on a good note. Ask your child this every single day and also answer yourself. Doing this may help you to learn something new about your child and their school, but perhaps even more importantly, it helps the mind to focus on something positive that is to come for the day rather than thinking about the negative or something that invokes worry.

How It Looks

Mornings often end up being full of rushing, running around, and sometimes yelling because no one wants to be late. Starting the day in this way can make for a stressful morning that may impact a negative mood. Whenever possible, getting things done the night ahead so that the morning can run more smoothly can support a less rushed morning. When asking your child about what they are looking forward to for the day, minimize distractions (turn off devices and music) and show that you are truly interested in their answer. You may ask them during breakfast while eating together, in the car on your way to school, or as they sit waiting for the bus.

Works Cited

Bishop, S. R., Lau, M., Shapiro, S., Carlson, L., Anderson, N. D., Carmody, J. ... Devins, G. (2004). Mindfulness: A proposed operational definition. *Clinical Psychology: Science and Practice, 11*(3), 230–241.

Smith Harvey, V. (2007, November). "Resiliency: Strategies for parents and educators." *National Association of School Psychologists (NASP).* www.nasponline.org/publications/periodicals/communique/issues/volume-36-issue-3/resiliency-strategies-for-parents-and-educators

Appendix A
Permission Form

I would like to invite _____ to participate in the *Using CBT and Mindfulness to Manage Anxiety* group. This group will utilize Cognitive-Behavioral Therapy (CBT) approaches and mindfulness practices. CBT includes the idea that our thoughts, feelings, and behaviors are all related and if we can understand the negative thoughts that arise and challenge these thoughts, we can then alter our feelings and behaviors. Mindfulness is a state of being in which we are aware of our thoughts and accepting of them in a way in which we don't feel a need to react or judge them. The focus of the group will be on supporting your child in reducing their worry while increasing their knowledge and use of coping strategies. Each session focuses on an awareness of our thinking and feelings. Your child will gain skills in recognizing their emotions; understanding the connection between our body, our thoughts, and our emotions; useful strategies in challenging negative thoughts; skills in evaluating problems to include consideration of what is in and outside of their control; an evaluation of relationships-considering people that are helpful or harmful to our inner thoughts; and an introduction of and practice of a variety of coping strategies.

Each week I will share a summary of the information your child learns with you. It would be especially helpful if you are able to check in with your child regarding their learning and model similar wording and strategies to help your child recognize our learning in action. Your support would be especially appreciated in providing positive reinforcement, "I noticed that you used a calming strategy when you were getting upset, I can tell you are making some great progress!"; and calmly offering supportive ideas when your child gets stuck, "I wonder if you are focusing on the worst-case scenario. What data do you have against this scenario, and as you think of that what is most likely to happen?" The more that your child is hearing this information, the more likely they are to internalize these practices and utilize them independently.

I plan to meet with your child (In a group/independently) _____ times per week for the next _____ weeks. During our time together, I will be gathering data about their progress and will share this data with you once our group is complete. For me to better understand your child's needs, I am asking for you to please complete the following Guardian Questionnaire. With your permission for this group, I will also have your child's teacher complete a similar form. This will help for each week's session to be customized to fit their unique needs.

Please reach out to me if you have any questions. I can be reached at
_____(phone) or _____(e-mail).

Thank you,

_____

Please mark one option below
[   ] I give my child permission to be a part of the *Learning to Cope with Worry* Group
[   ] I do not give my child permission to be a part of the *Learning to Cope with Worry* Group

_____   _____
(Signature)   (Date)

Appendix B-G

Guardian Questionnaire

Thank you for agreeing to have your child join me as we work together in learning to cope with worry. Since you know your child best, I would appreciate if you were able to complete the following questions and send them back to school with your child for our first meeting on _____ (date). If you have any questions, please don't hesitate to reach out.

This form is being filled out by _____ (your name) regarding

_____ (child's name)

1   What I love best about my child is….

2   My child most worries about….

3   My child often exhibits these physical symptoms which may be related to worry (Circle all that apply)

Stomach Pain	Headache	Racing Heart	Body Constantly Moving
Clenched Jaw	Sweaty Hands	Darting Eyes	Other:

4   My child has experienced a panic attack – Yes/No/Unsure (Circle one)
   * If yes, please provide further information about this experience:

5   My child has experienced trauma – Yes/No/Unsure (Circle one)
   * If yes, please provide further information about their trauma.

6 Strategies that help my child when they are feeling worried are:

7 Strategies that do not help my child when they are feeling worried are:

8 Something that is important for you to know about my child is….

9 A goal I have for my child during their time working on worries is….

Thank you for your time in completing this survey. Please return with your child to school

Attn: _____ (Practitioner's name)

Sincerely,

_____ (Practitioner's name)

_____ (Phone Number)

_____ (E-mail address)

Appendix B-T
Teacher Questionnaire

Thank you for allowing your student to join me as we work together in learning to cope with worry. Since you see your student more frequently than I do throughout the week, I would appreciate if you were able to complete the following questions and return them to me by _____ (Date). If you have any questions, please don't hesitate to reach out.

This form is being filled out by _____ (your name) regarding

_____ (student's name)

1 My favorite thing about this student is….

2 I most notice that this student appears worried by…

3 My student often exhibits these physical symptoms which may be related to worry (Circle all that apply)

Stomach Pain	Headache	Racing Heart	Body Constantly Moving
Clenched Jaw	Sweaty Hands	Darting Eyes	Other:

4 This student excels in _____ at school.

5 This student struggles most with _____ at school.

6 Describe your student's interactions with peers.

7 What calming strategies have you introduced in the classroom? Which of these are most preferred by the student?

8 Something that is important for you to know about this student is...

9 A goal I have for this student while working on their worries is...

Thank you for your time in completing this survey. Please return to

_____ (Practitioner's name)

Sincerely,

_____ (Practitioner's name)

_____ (Phone Number)

_____ (e-mail address)

Appendix C
Pre-Post Test

	Not at All		Somewhat		All the Time
When I start to worry, my mind can't stop thinking*	◯	◯	◯	◯	◯
I notice when I feel worry within my body	◯	◯	◯	◯	◯
I know how to calm my body when I feel worried	◯	◯	◯	◯	◯
I know how challenge my thoughts	◯	◯	◯	◯	◯
I know of different ways to help myself feel calm.	◯	◯	◯	◯	◯

*Reverse score this item

Appendix D

Weakly Assessment

	Not at All		Somewhat		All the Time
This week I have felt worried...*	◯	◯	◯	◯	◯
I recognize different emotions I am feeling during the day.	◯	◯	◯	◯	◯
This week I was able to calm my body when I felt worried.	◯	◯	◯	◯	◯

Reverse score this item

Appendix E

Emotions Worksheet

Emotion	Time you felt this Emotion	My body felt...	My mind was thinking...
Sad			
Excited			
Worried			
Happy			
Frustrated			
Shame			

Appendix F-A

Deep Breathing Choices for Adolescents

4-7-8 Breathing	• Breathe in for a count of 4 • Hold for a count of 7 • Breathe out for a count of 8
5-4-3-2-1 Grounding	• Take a deep breath in through your nose and out through your mouth, name 5 things you can see • Take a deep breath in through your nose and out through your mouth, name 4 things you can touch • Take a deep breath in through your nose and out through your mouth, name 3 things you can hear • Take a deep breath in through your nose and out through your mouth, name 2 things you can smell • Take a deep breath in through your nose and out through your mouth, name 1 thing you can taste
Shoulder Breathing 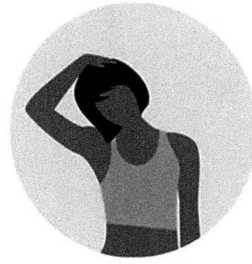	• Grab your right ear with your left hand and gently pull your head toward your left shoulder. Take three deep breaths in and out • Grab your left ear with your right hand and gently pull your head toward your right shoulder. Take three deep breaths in and out

Appendix F-C
Deep Breathing Choices for Children

4-7-8 Breathing 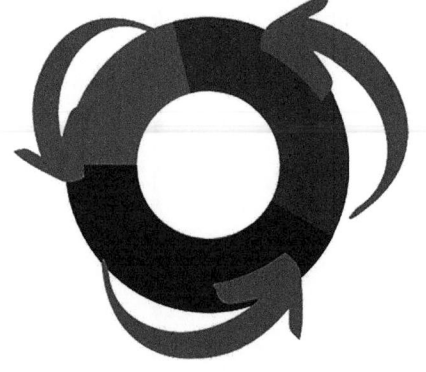	• Breathe in for a count of 4 • Hold for a count of 7 • Breathe out for a count of 8
Finger Breathing 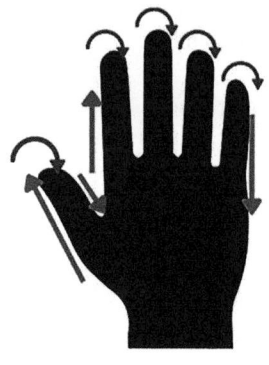	• Hold one hand out with fingers open and take the opposite hand's pointer finger. • Trace the open hand by starting on the outside by the thumb. • Take your pointer finger up to the top of the thumb and breathe in, and then breathe out while going down the opposite side of your thumb. • Continue this motion breathing in when going up the next finger and then out when going down until you've traced all the fingers.
Belly Breathing 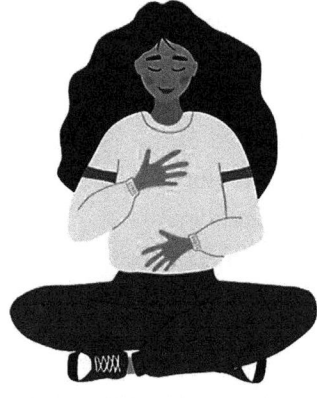	• Hold your hand on your stomach and slowly breathe in through your nose (feeling your hand rise as your belly expands) • Then slowly breathe out and feel your belly shrink back

Appendix G

Worry Sheet

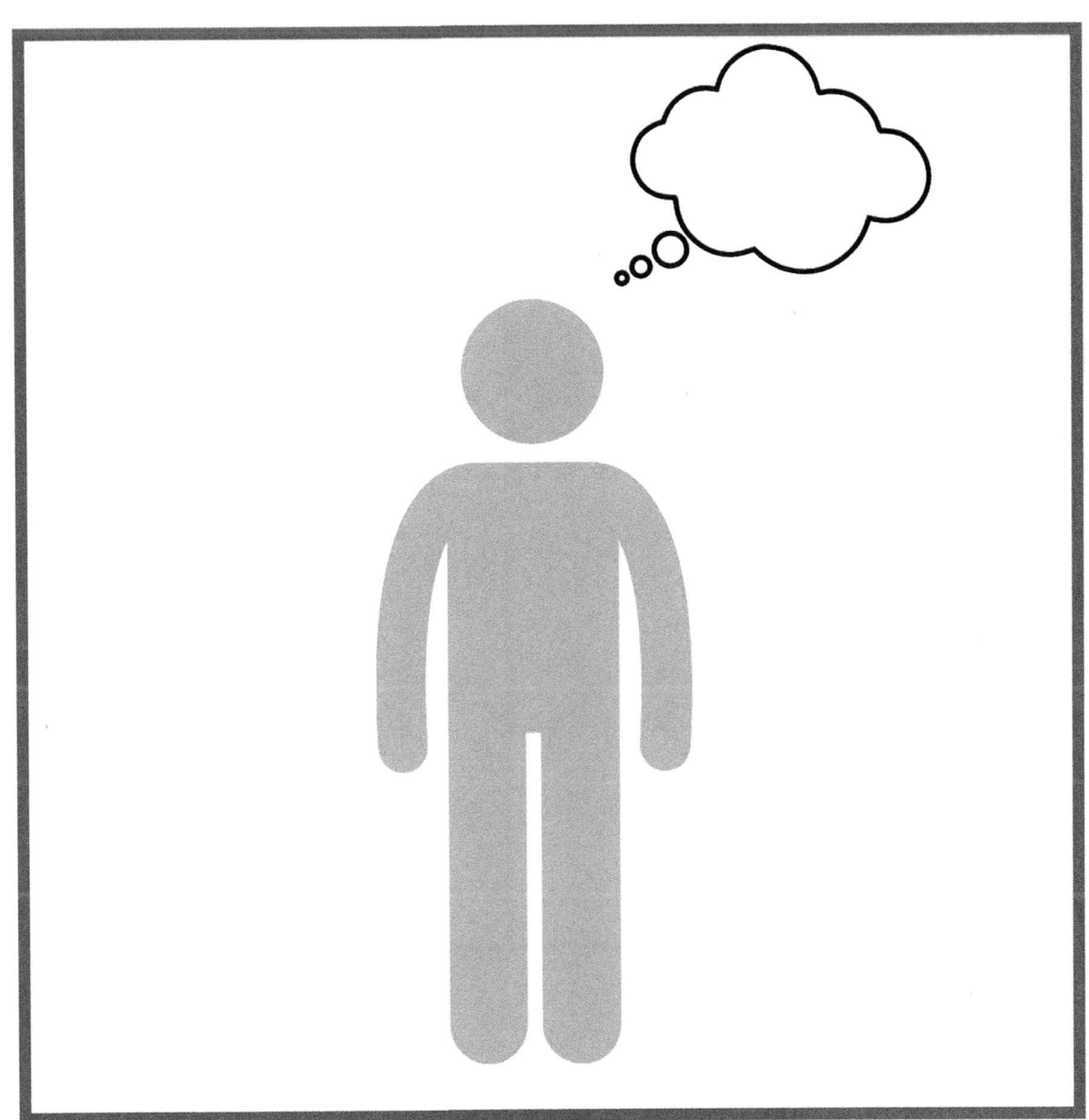

<u>What Stopped the Worry?</u>

Appendix H.1
Thought Reframing – Most Likely Scenario

Explain your situation of worry

What is the worst case scenario?	What evidence do you have against the worst case happening?	What is the best case scenario?	What is most likely to happen?

Appendix H.2

Thought Reframing – Possible Options

Explain your situation of worry

Possible Option	Possible Outcome	Level of anxiety	Ability to manage worry
		5 4 3 2 1	
		5 4 3 2 1	
		5 4 3 2 1	
		5 4 3 2 1	

Circle the option that would make the best choice for you

Appendix I

Control and Stress

Identify the Problem

What is within your control? (Playdoh)	What is outside of your control? (Rock)

Examples:
  ○ Your actions - how you respond
  ○ Calming your body and mind
	Examples:
	  ○ Other people's actions
	  ○ Something that has already happened

Appendix J
Coping Strategies

What my body needs	Activity	I would try this
Movement	Yoga	Yes - Maybe. - No
	Walking	Yes - Maybe. - No
	Running	Yes - Maybe. - No
	Sports	Yes - Maybe. - No
	Weightlifting	Yes - Maybe. - No
	Fidgeting with a Sensory Object	Yes - Maybe. - No
	Riding a Bike	Yes - Maybe. - No
Creativity	Drawing	Yes - Maybe. - No
	Coloring	Yes - Maybe. - No
	Journaling	Yes - Maybe. - No
	Taking Pictures	Yes - Maybe. - No
	Organizing a Space	Yes - Maybe. - No
	Listening to music	Yes - Maybe. - No
	Cooking or Baking	Yes - Maybe. - No
Stillness	Mindful Meditation – App	Yes - Maybe. - No
	Mindful Breathing – App	Yes - Maybe. - No
	5-4-3-2-1 Grounding	Yes - Maybe. - No
	Deep Breathing Tool	Yes - Maybe. - No
	Progressive Muscle Relaxation	Yes - Maybe. - No
	Reading	Yes - Maybe. - No
	Resting	Yes - Maybe. - No
Gratitude	Writing 3 Things You're Thankful For	Yes - Maybe. - No
	Writing 3 Things you Love about Yourself	Yes - Maybe. - No
	Writing a Thank You Note	Yes - Maybe. - No
	Doing Something Kind for Someone	Yes - Maybe. - No
Connection	Getting a Hug	Yes - Maybe. - No
	Asking for Help	Yes - Maybe. - No
	Smiling and Laughing with Someone	Yes - Maybe. - No
	Cuddling a Pet	Yes - Maybe. - No
	Talking to an Adult	Yes - Maybe. - No
	Talking to a Friend	Yes - Maybe. - No

Appendix K

Positive/Negative Influences and Relationships

What makes me, me?	What behaviors do I enjoy being around?	What behaviors bother me when being around others?

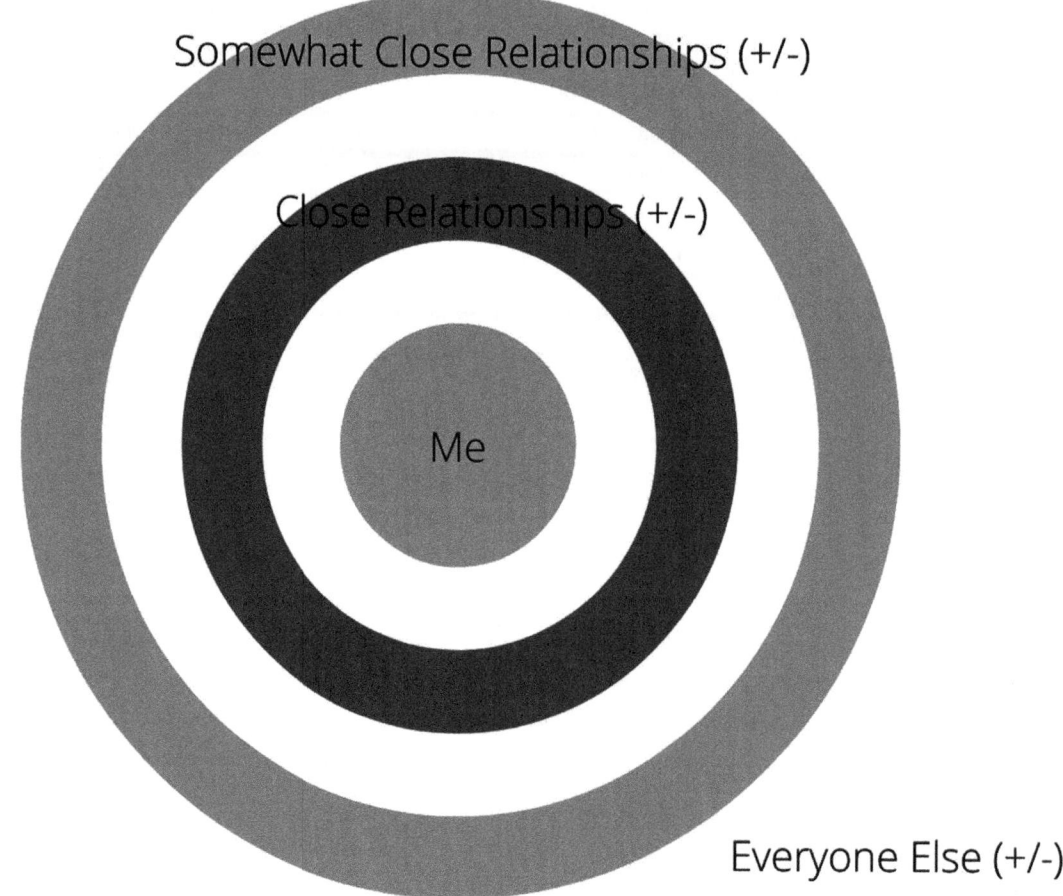

Somewhat Close Relationships (+/-)

Close Relationships (+/-)

Me

Everyone Else (+/-)

Appendix L
Calm Strategy Rating

Mindful Meditation - Progressive Muscle Relaxation Exercise

	Tense		Somewhat Calm		Very Calm
The feeling of my body is...	○	○	○	○	○
The feeling of my mind is...	○	○	○	○	○

Yoga - Tree Pose

	Tense		Somewhat Calm		Very Calm
The feeling of my body is...	○	○	○	○	○
The feeling of my mind is...	○	○	○	○	○

Creativity - Drawing/ Coloring/ Journaling

	Tense		Somewhat Calm		Very Calm
The feeling of my body is...	○	○	○	○	○
The feeling of my mind is...	○	○	○	○	○

Gratitude - Reflection of gratitude for three things

	Tense		Somewhat Calm		Very Calm
The feeling of my body is...	○	○	○	○	○
The feeling of my mind is..	○	○	○	○	○

Appendix M
Calming Practice

Date:	
How was I feeling?	
What practice did I try?	
How did I feel afterward?	

Date:	
How was I feeling?	
What practice did I try?	
How did I feel afterward?	

Date:	
How was I feeling?	
What practice did I try?	
How did I feel afterward?	

Appendix N
Student Worry Plan

I can recognize I am starting to feel worried by paying attention to my body and mind	
This happens in my body…	This happens in my mind…

When I am worried, others may recognize me doing this…

When I am feeling worried the following things can help (Circle what works for you)

Go for a walk	Paint	Listen to a mindful meditation practice	Talk with someone
Practice yoga	Draw	Choose a deep breathing exercise	Write in a journal
Go for a run	Organize something	5-4-3-2-1 Breathing	Pet an animal
Weightlifting	Coloring	Dancing	Other:

If the strategies I try on my own don't work, these people can help me when I am feeling worried…

Person 1 at home:		Person 1 at School:	
Person 2 at home:		Person 2 at School:	

This person can help by… (Circle what will work for you)

Talking me through Worst/Best/Most likely scenario	Joining me in a calming strategy	Walking with me	Talking me through what is within and outside of my control
Helping me find a quiet space	Coloring/drawing with me	Allowing me to journal	Other:

It is not helpful when someone…

I will know I am feeling better by paying attention to my body and mind	
This is how my body will feel…	This is how my mind will feel…

Index

Note: *Italicized*, **bold** and ***bold italics*** refer to figures, tables and boxes, respectively.

accommodations 113–114
adolescents: anxiety in 1–4; deep breathing choices for 139; emotions in 42, 44, 45; emotions with feelings in body and thoughts, integrating 48–51; worry in 1–4
anxiety: in adolescents 1–4; behavioral symptoms of 3; in children 1–4; cognitive symptoms of 3; distinguished from worry 2–3; generalized 4; physical symptoms of 2–3; separation 4; social 4; somatic symptoms of 4
automatic thoughts 7, 8, 11–14, 24–26

Baer, R. A. 23
Bartram, D. 17
behavioral symptoms of anxiety/worry 3
behaviors 8–10
body: emotions with feelings in, integrating 47–53
Boschet, J. M. 3
Breath Awareness 105, ***106***
breathing: breathe in positivity 112, *112*; breathe out negativity 112, *112*; deep 110; and mindfulness 22; square 111, *111*

calming 79–84, 94; practice 148
calm space: classroom 101–103, *102*; home *120*, 121–122
calm strategy rating 147
CBT *see* cognitive behavioral therapy (CBT)
Chand, S. P. 7, 8
children: anxiety in 1–4; deep breathing choices for 140; emotions in 41–45; emotions with feelings in body and thoughts, integrating 48, 51–52; worry in 1–4
Classroom Intention 104, ***105***
cognitive behavioral therapy (CBT) 7–19; behaviors 8–10; coping strategies 17–19; emotions 8–10; mindfulness and *see* mindfulness; within and out of control 15–16; reframing thoughts 10–15; thoughts 8–10
cognitive distortions 7–8, 11, 12, 24, 25
cognitive symptoms of anxiety/worry 3
control: in and out of 65–70; within and out of 15–16; and stress 144
coping: emotion-focused 17; problem-focused 17; strategies 17–19, 65–70, 79–84, 91–95, 145
creativity, and mindfulness 22

daily mindfulness 104–108
deep breathing 110; choices, for adolescents 139; choices, for children 140

emotion-focused coping 17
emotions 8–10; acceptance of 24–26; in adolescents 42, 44, 45; awareness 23; check-in 98–100, *99*; in children 41–45; with feelings in body and thoughts, integrating 47–53; worksheet 138
empowerment 2

family mindfulness 123–124

Gardner, D. 17
generalized anxiety 4
Gluck, V. M. 3
gratitude reflection 118, **119**
guardian questionnaire 131, 132–133

Huecker, M. R. 7, 8

IEP *see* Individualized Education Plan (IEP)
Individualized Education Plan (IEP): goals 115
informal practice, and mindfulness 23

Kuckel, D. P. 7, 8

Larson, R. W. 11
Loving-Kindness Meditation 107–108, *108*

MBIs *see* mindfulness-based interventions (MBIs)
Minahan, J. 3
Mindful Moments 109, **109**
mindfulness 21–27; benefits of 21; breath work and 22; creativity and 22; daily 104–108; definition of 21; family 123–124; informal practice and 23; movement and 22; practices, for students 23–27; visualization and 22–23
mindfulness-based interventions (MBIs) 23
Mindful Walking 107, ***107***
movement, and mindfulness 22

negative thoughts, changing 55–63

Orson, C. N. 11

permission form 131
phobia 4
physical symptoms of anxiety/worry 2–3
Pittig, A. 3
planning 127
Play-Doh problems 65–70
Positive Moment Visualization 106, *106*
positive/negative influences 146
positive thinking 126
praise 127
pre-post test 136
problem-focused coping 17

Rappaport, N. 3
rapport, building 33–39
reframing thoughts 10–15, 24–26; most likely
    scenario 142; possible options 143
relationships 71–77, 146
resiliency 1–2

Sauer, S. 23
Schneider, K. 3
separation anxiety 4

social anxiety 4
somatic symptoms of anxiety 4
square breathing 110, *111*
Stanton, A. L. 17
stress, control and 144
stress reduction practices 79–84
students: mindfulness practices for 23–27; plan
    85–90; rapport, building 33–39; selection 29;
    worry plan 149

Taylor, S. E. 17
teacher questionnaire 134–135
thoughts 8–10; acceptance of 24–26;
    emotions with feelings in, integrating
    47–53; negative, changing 55–63; reframing
    10–15, 24–26, 142–143

underlying beliefs 7

visualization: and mindfulness 22–23; Positive
    Moment Visualization 106, *106*

weekly assessment 137
worry **36**; in adolescents 1–4; behavioral symptoms
    of 3; box 125; in children 1–4; cognitive symptoms
    of 3; definition of 2; distinguished from anxiety
    2–3; physical symptoms of 2–3; sheet 141